My Health and Fitness

Volume 2

I0420076

47 Articles

By: Wade Yoder

Master Trainer - Fitness Nutrition Specialist

- Health & Fitness Columnist

Introduction

Does the constant barrage of advertisements for weight loss, anti-aging strategies, and chronic disease scare tactics make you want clarity and simplicity? If it does you have enter into an area of unison with your body. Our body wants the simple things with consistency, this is how we overcome chronic disease, premature aging, obesity, mobility problems and get into the best shape of our life!

Example: our immune system is made strong by healthy habits; it is made nimble by exposure to our surroundings. Keeping from exposing our immune system to pathogens so it doesn't struggle is like saying a muscle is better off without resistance. Our body adapts to adversity and becomes stronger because of it; all it asks of us is simple healthy habits in consistent daily doses.

My Health and Fitness Volume 2 is a mix of 47 articles on burning body fat naturally, building muscle without supplements, increasing mobility and capability, prevention of chronic disease and premature aging. These fundamentals have not changed and the confusion fear and hype surrounding them is not for your benefit. I have been in the health club business since 1991 and have seen a lot of fads and hype come and go, but not without taking a lot of our money with them.

I believe in reverse diagnostics and that by using this approach it will help us to find the root cause of our problem. When we correct the root problem, we no longer have to medicate its symptom(s).

When it comes to our health, fitness, mobility issues and our capability to prevent chronic disease **we should always see how many questions we can ask ourselves about our area of concern.** We too often ask ones who have mixed alliances and their answers are distorted due to personal gain…

Dedicated to: the discouraged, the scared, the financially strapped, the hurting, the confused, the frustrated and last but not least, the ones who feel that spending a major amount of their life in doctor's office waiting rooms and endless diagnosis's is the new norm...

This book and series is dedicated to helping everyone I can to realize the power of the body's own resources when given the simple basics that it craves, such as the body's capability to fight premature aging and chronic disease, by formulating its own drugs through the power of the immune system.

Health, fitness, muscle building and weight loss should not be looked at as something that costs a lot of money. Our health and fitness is adaptive to the habits we adopt.

If this book helps make your path to health and fitness an easier less complicated one, then my mission is accomplished~ Wade Yoder

Table of Contents

DON'T BE ASHAMED OF YOUR NEW YEAR'S RESOLUTIONS!

Making New Year's health and fitness resolutions is not something to be ashamed of, it is however something to worry about if we no longer place any value on them, especially when we know we need to change our physical condition and if we at all believe there may be some value to decreasing our dependence on the medical healthcare system!

When we no longer have enough of that burning desire to change something that needs changing, (by creating a personal resolve within ourselves to make this change), we are then accepting ourselves in a way that usually does not stay the same, but simply continues to get worse. This often leads to a dependence on others, (when in all reality they have no reason to care more for our health then we do). Have you ever helped someone and noticed that they cared less then you did? Doesn't make you feel like helping anymore, right?

When we make these health and fitness goals, we probably don't realize at the end of the year how many times it has actually helped us in avoiding those extra pieces of dessert, those extra walks, the extra 15 min added to our workouts etc. We may not have come close to the lofty fitness goal we set, and what we wanted to look and feel like by the end of the year, BUT if we could see what we avoided looking and feeling like, it would be enough to inspire us at the turn of the next year! These things really accumulate either way you choose to go.

Example: someone can choose to skip sweet drinks and desserts for a year or someone can make the subconscious choice to continue consuming them for a year and this could make a huge difference between weight gained vs. weight lost. Dessert, soda's, sweet tea etc. added into a meal can easily make up an extra 250 calories in one meal.

250 calories x 365 days in a year = 91,250 extra calories and it only takes 3,500 calories to build a pound of fat. That's an extra 26 pounds of potential fat. Even if we only gain half of that, its still an extra 13 pounds and if we don't stop it, within 3 years, we will have gained 39 pounds and within 10 years this can turn into a morbidly overweight issue when we are carrying an extra 130 pounds on a frame and system that is simply not built to sustain that kind of weight.

It works exactly the opposite if we make these small healthy choices and it can also really accumulate over the course of a year, if we can change what we think tastes good and feels good to our body and make our decisions based on how it will make us feel an hour from now, tomorrow, next month or a year from now!

A calendar can be a great accountability partner by simply writing in our goal for the following December, then writing in our weekly, monthly, quarterly assessments of our progress. Writing in our progress or a lack there of, can be encouraging even if the notes and assessments do not make us feel good!

Some Simple Steps for the new year: avoid sugary food and drink, exercise whether skinny, fat, or in-between (this helps us push out the bad things that cause disease), avoid packaged and fast foods, (eat healthy one item ingredients such as vegetables, fruits, nuts, eggs, berries, quality lean meats and dairy, and beans), get deep rest, avoid stress or at least learn to de-stress, educate yourself a little every day on health and fitness issues, stay active and fill in non-active days with a good exercise routine.

Each year we have the God given capability for a completely new cell generation, and the healthy habits we adopt now is what helps our present generation of cells have healthier baby cells!

We are not an island and our healthy choices have more of a ripple effect then we oft times think! Lets make our new year a healthy year for ourselves and the ones we care about!

Our health and fitness habits today will be our currency tomorrow!

IMMUNE SYSTEM FITNESS VS. INFLUENZA

Our immune system works 24-7-365 and knows

exactly what's wrong with us and what it needs to

repair it with, whether its better food to work with,

more water, more rest, less stress, or more exercise.

The immune system gets stronger first by getting

depressed. It's like muscle fibers that have been

broken down during a really hard workout. Our
body uses this signal to build the muscle back
stronger, to prepare it to handle the physical stress
that we have told it that it can start expecting from
us. If we workout too hard when we first start
exercising or when our body is not fully recovered
from the previous exercise routine, we increase the
risk or injury and if the injury is bad enough it can
put us out of commission for a while. Strengthening
our immune system works much the same way, in
how that it strengthens itself through exposures to

our surroundings. Just like muscle, if we live in a sterilized bubble for long enough, our immune system will waste away, since it never gets exercised.

Most of us have at one time or the other ate and exercised to get in a certain condition, whether it was taking in more protein to build muscle, or dropping sugar and starch intake to drop body fat levels. Building our immune system works in much the same way, healthy balanced diet, exercise, plenty of rest and let's not forget, exposure on a

consistent basis to your environment strengthens our immune system naturally. And just like over doing it when exercising, we can also over do it when exposing ourselves to our surrounding environment when we know we are feeling run down. When we already feel run down, it's the wrong time to expose ourselves to potential pathogens.

Important things we can do to strengthen and keep our immune system strong:

1. Deep rest and plenty of it, this is when our body repairs itself

2. Drink plenty of water. Try to drink at least 12-16 oz. upon waking; this will help your body eliminate things it wants to get out of you. Lemon squeezed into warm water in the morning is a good immune booster, along with many other benefits!

3. Plenty of antioxidant and mineral rich vegetables, fruits, nuts & berries should be in your diet, this helps the several trillion cells in our body have a better defense system. If you do not get enough of these, use vitamins & minerals (backed with scientific research and not hype) to supplement your diet. Remember, food in balance is your best source of nutrients.

4. Try to prevent breathing sudden blast of cold air, when leaving a temperature controlled environment, a simple dust mask works well, or pulling jacket, shirt or scarf over your nose.

5. Stay active and exercise, but if you feel run down, layoff or at least do not exercise strenuously, your body does not need to be fighting the flu and trying to recover from a workout.

6. When you or the ones you care about are going to be around crowds of people or an environment that may increase your risk, be sure to keep yourself as healthy as you can leading up to the exposure.

When your immune system is tired, it's simply a lot harder to fight off the bad things around us.

7. Avoid stress and if you do get stressed, find something you enjoy doing to de-stress, such as active sports, reading, a funny movie, meditation etc.

8. Think healthy thoughts about yourself and your health, it can have some pretty cool and positive benefits when your brain/control center of your body is kept positive!

We've got a powerful system within us that is constantly sending alert signals and gathering defenses to kill foreign invaders as they enter our body, but if we do not give it the (simple healthy basics) to build the weaponry it needs, it will lose its battles and when our immune system is not working properly, we begin to lose quality of life and capability to fight illness and disease.

Our immune system takes our health more serious then anyone else on this planet, are we willing to give it the tools it needs to keep us well?

Side note: when a publication, media or the medical professional is pushing immunization through laboratory created vaccines and medicine for flu prevention and chronic disease and they omit the healthy basic habits that build our immune system naturally, I personally feel they are motivated by wealth created through medicating disease and are much more concerned about their wealth then my health.

We must ask ourselves, why are flu viruses, and chronic diseases seeming to get worse with more complicated mutations every year along with the ensuing widespread dependence on sick care? Are we forgetting that our immune system can learn and sequence an invader better then any external guesswork can? The immune system is the ONLY thing that actually heals us.

THE PLANK ...GREAT FOR PROTECTING YOUR BACK!

Our back/spine (besides helping with all sorts of upper body movements such as twisting, turning, stretching, bending) is like a pipe that holds the hardwiring for our different body parts, whether it's vital organs involuntary actions or our skeletal movement. If our back is not strengthened and properly protected and something mashes the casing that holds your nerves it can cause all sorts of problems.

Example: if wiring gets severed or grounded out that supplies a subdivision with power, this could effect all the different houses in that particular grid, so it would be very important to the power company to keep the supply line protected from the elements so as to provide uninterrupted power and signal going into this area. It is much more important that we protect this part of our central nervous system, (the spine).

The Plank: the plank is an exercise that you can do almost anywhere and no equipment is necessary. This is a static exercise (also known as isometric and will affect muscles at high intensities without joint movement).

This affects the core area of the body (abdominals), and is an area that most of us would like to shape anyhow. This gets muscles all around the core and does not just focus on one area like crunches and sit-ups do. Exercising only one side of our core can cause muscle imbalance. The best way that I can describe a muscle imbalance is to compare it to hanging a weight off of one side of a bicycle instead of balancing the weight evenly with both sides. We know what will happen if we try to ride the bike, it will keep trying to pull us in the direction of where most of the weight is hanging on. This is much how fat and muscle work, if its not evenly distributed and it will eventually cause a strain on our skeletal structure because of the pull in that direction. This can also lead to a degenerative condition in these areas and can lead up to the point that a doctor will try to convince you to repair it through surgery, or at the least a chiropractor for a long series of decompression treatments. We can avoid a lot of potential injury and increase our quality of life by staying consistent with a few exercises that only take a small amount of time but could prevent some big problems later.

How to do the Plank: lie facedown on the floor with your body straight and your forearms resting on the floor. Slowly press your body up off the floor onto your forearms and toes. Keep your abs pulled in tight and your back flat while holding this position. It is something almost anyone can do for a few seconds and when done with consistency you will find that you can hold the position for longer.

The neat thing is this: whenever muscular strength or endurance is increased, you can feel good about this area being not only stronger but better protected with muscle support. This is your way of surrounding a wore down skeletal area of the body a natural splint.

This is very important when launching a fitness routine as well. All the bouncing around that we do when we first start out can cause compression and inflammation around nerves and when this happens, it can put a lot of pressure on the area along with potential inflammation flare-ups, and besides the pain and aggravation, it can also make so the signal that our brain is trying to send out to different parts of our body do not reach their destination properly.

Our back and neck should be looked at as one of our most guarded investments, since it is through these that the brain sends its messages whether voluntary or involuntary for almost all of our life functions. Whether for prevention of back problems or strengthening a weak one, less then 3 minutes a day could make a big difference!

THE COLOR OF FITNESS

If you have a special day coming up and want to look your best for the ones in your life and for the pictures that freeze us in time, here are a few shape-up tips for the countdown to your special day!

Diet: it is very important to eat a wide variety of colors in our diet if we want that healthy glow and it can be pretty easy if we simply surround ourselves with a rainbow of colors (these colors are different nutrients) in our fruit and vegetable selections. This blend of colors is what gives us a healthy glow on the outside and it also reflects what is going on inside! Note; skittles don't do the same thing! Taking in plenty of fruits and vegetables during this time also helps our body get rid of the toxins that have built up throughout our body in a safe manner. Try to keep intake at about 75% vegetables and 25% fruits, especially for weight loss. Also fruits in the morning help assist in the daily detox time period after waking, so fruits in the morning and vegetables for lunch and dinner. Making sure you have good sources of protein helps insure muscle recovery from strenuous workouts and keeping good fats/oils in your diet help keep things running smoothly and helps keep skin lustrous. When we lose too much of the subcutaneous fat that is under the skin, it can make our skin look old.

Tricking your body into burning fat: when you drop your food/caloric intake really low for one or two days, it forces your body to seek alternative fuel and it simply opens the trap doors on your fat cells and lets energy out. The problem with doing this for too long comes in when you hit about the 3rd day and your body thinks you don't have an adequate supply of food to supply all your muscular energy needs, so it simply starts burning off some muscle so it can slow your metabolism down. So don't do real low calorie for more then two days and if you go for a complete fast or Intermittent Fasting (IF) go for only 18-24 hours. When you have your up-calorie day, your body will send the calories straight to your muscle and vital organs, and if you eat in excess of your needs, only then will it restock your fat cells. I like this for the speed of dropping weight without a lot of muscle loss.

The Shape Up: muscle tones, shapes and builds by first being broke down from exertion it's not used to. When it recovers, it builds back stronger, more toned, shaped and capable to handle the new stress that you have been putting this particular set of muscles under! This is your opportunity to sculpt the areas you want to! If done with consistency, (along with increasing the resistance or the number of repetitions), it can really make a difference in a short amount of time!

Keep your routine simple and stick with exercises that get multiple muscles, such as, the Bench Press or Pushups for chest and back of arms (triceps) - Rowing exercises (such as cable row or bent row with dumbbells) for the back and front of arms (biceps) - and squats or lunges for legs. Picking one exercise from the above gets most of the major muscle groups and each group gets to rest while you're working on the next one in the circuit. This keeps the heart rate up which will trigger the process that burns fat for energy. If you do not have time for the above and need something very effective to do at home, you can do an exercise that gets most of your muscles with a single movement.

Take a set of dumbbells, spread your feet, drop into a full squat touching dumbbells at floor beside your ankles, come back up rapidly pressing dumbbells up overhead, do a few warm-up reps and then do a minimum of 2-3 sets to exhaustion. Do this every other day and consider this your sculpting day, the next day simply do some cardio such as rapid pace walking for about 30 minutes. Remember that the speed the reps and routine are executed, not only increase intensity for toning purposes but it also speeds fat loss!

There is something about a person that has a healthy look coming out through their skin and eyes that exudes an energetic magnetism that is sexy and attractive to your spouse even if at a larger size. So whatever the size is that we feel is right for us, attaining this without inner health will strike down the appeal of a reduced size.

RAPID AND EXPLOSIVE MOVEMENT

There are several ways that we can increase the intensity of an exercise to stimulate further development of muscle, bone, tendon and ligament strength.

1. We can increase the weight or resistance, so that the targeted muscle group has to work harder lifting, pulling, pressing or pushing a weight.

2. We can also move the same weight we have been using faster creating a greater resistance on the muscles being used. When we move the same amount of weight through the same distance at a faster speed, (weird as it may sound), it increases the resistance and forces the muscle to work harder, thus stimulating the muscle group to adapt to this new intensity. The first one is a method that is used most times in a gym, but when someone has a more limited amount of equipment or weights at home, (such as using one's bodyweight for exercises), the second way can be a good way to move around the limitations restricting workout intensity, simply by doing the movement faster. You can also intensify a walking routine by not only walking rapidly, but also stopping every 5 minutes and doing a rapid set of 10-15 squats.

This is a big part of why programs such as P90X have worked so well for ones that have stuck it out and why the ones doing it have a more muscular and sculpted shape vs. results one oft time sees coming from such things as conventional aerobic classes, treadmills, jogging, steppers, and elliptical machines. A good example would be the leg development of a high-speed short distance runner vs. a long distance runner.

Since working muscles require blood and oxygen, rapid or explosive movement of especially the large muscle groups will increase the need for blood and oxygen, this is why our heart rate and breathing will speed up so as to meet the demand. If this demand is kept up for approximately 20 minutes or longer it will send a signal to meet another need, this time it will be for energy. This is when our fat cells start releasing their energy and we get to the fat burn zone, (known as our 2nd wind).

We need to gradually work our way up to avoid injury. Our body adapts to new demands placed on it, whether its our muscle, bones, tendons, ligaments, brain or even our immune system, but if we place to much demand and without adequate recovery we can increase risk of injury same as in over exposure of our immune system can lead to illness.

Take away: whether its pushups, in place bodyweight squats, a walk or a regular workout in a gym, we can increase the intensity of our workout by keeping an eye on the clock and gradually pushing ourselves to do the same amount in a shorter amount of time. This works as well at any job at the work place that requires physical output. We can turn our (housework, construction site, walking from car to work, taking stairs etc.) into an exercise routine by increasing speed of movement. Remember to fuel your engine with water first thing every morning, (its the next thing in line of importance to oxygen), and it does so much physiologically in the body, it should be called "gym-in-a-bottle!"

Rapid and explosive movement develops more muscle, burns more calories, and it gets more done in a shorter amount of time, whether in work or in our workouts!

TOXIC BELLY FAT...A POISON FUEL!

Fat has many good purposes (one of the main ones being our backup energy source), but one kind of fat that can be very bad for our shape and our health, is visceral fat that has turned toxic! Though fat storage is a vital source of energy, if it becomes toxic, it can also become an energy source for disease.

Visceral fat is the fat that builds up around the waist area and can gradually thickly surround vital organs such as your liver, intestines, kidneys and your stomach. I like to imagine visceral fat as surrounding our plumbing (vital organs etc.) with an energy insulation that can also absorb toxins that stay in our system, when they don't get flushed out through normal elimination, such as (sweating, urination and bowel movement). Once this fat gets very toxic, (even for a thin person) its sort of like an over soaked sponge that sets there secreting poisonous inflammatory toxins into our organs and tissues, that can lead to organ failure and other chronic diseases with names attached, once the inflammation has manifested itself into a discoverable and nameable disease.

Visceral fat as well as any other fat is a storage area for energy and back in the hunter-gatherer days provided a quick source of energy when needed whether it was in fight or flight. The hormones we secrete into our systems when we're scared, tensed up, or stressed out encourages even more visceral fat storage around our midsection for the purpose of reserve energy. A big difference is now we have plenty of stress but very little fight and flight to burn off these fat calories (from the visceral fat storage) and also to return our stress hormones back to normal. Cortisol is a stress hormone and a major culprit in directing the body to store belly fat. (Much of this can be offset by regular exercise and other means of lowering stress levels).

Quite possibly, many of the health problems we are having today is due in big part to not only the wrong calories and too many of them, but also our body's system constantly being flooded with hormones (such as adrenaline and cortisol) from constantly being on red alert, with no follow up of fight, flight, or exercise to relieve this angst with the good feel hormones that come with high energy expenditure, such as the feel good endorphins. We have an abundance of mental stress oft times without getting physically stressed afterwards, which is a good way to work off the former.

We are constantly bombarded with toxins in the air, foods etc. and unless our body has a consistent way to get it out, it will simply insulate the toxin in fat or mucous for our protection. Even a thin person can have visceral fat that has turned toxic from years of environmental exposures combined with poor dietary choices and a lack of intense physical activity. A lot of the toxicities that stay in our system, are due to the types of food and drink in our diets that simply do not encourage elimination of these, and when we constantly have stress hormones circulating in our system directing fat storage around the midsection, (we not only have a lot of unnecessary energy storage in this area) we also have a potentially big toxic sponge that sets there entwined around our organs soaking up and then releasing bad chemicals that cause inflammation, which is the root of almost all chronic disease!

The body tries to hang on to fat when it's trying to protect us from these toxins, and since mucous and fat surround these things to protect us, if we can simply detoxify our body we take away the reason stubborn fat is stubborn. This takes time and keeping protective micronutrients (from fruits and vegetables) going through our system helps assure safe release of these toxins and likewise the safe release of fat.

What we can do:

1. 3-5 hours of moderate to rapid pace activity per week, "this not only will help burn off the visceral fat around our midsections, but will also help in working off the stress that is telling our body to put it there! Any rapid activity can constitute as exercise, so get creative by having a mix of things you enjoy, such as hiking, biking, jogging, swimming, tennis etc. along with consistent weight bearing exercises to keep everything strong. Workup a good sweat at least 3 times a week, this helps push toxins out.

2. Increase water and fiber intake to help eliminate toxins. We should take in 1/2 our body weight in ounces of water minimum and at least 5 grams of fiber per serving for anything that goes in our mouth except for protein and water, (fiber binds up and carries out toxins & water flushes).

3. At least 5 servings of fruits and vegetables daily, "this keeps our antioxidant levels high in the blood and helps our body to get rid of the toxins circulating in our systems that cause aging and disease.

4. Find whatever means you can to de-stress your life, do everything you can to get good quality sleep, this is when our body recovers from the stresses of daily living!

Mental stress is a BIG cause of two things...belly fat and death!

A VALENTINE YOUR HEART
CAN FEEL

I'm sure that most of us have or will experience a time period in February when we absolutely wished we could press the vaporize button on the week of the 14th or at least that things could be better leading up to this day!

The month of February is considered American Heart Month, so I thought we would draw some correlation between the similarities in all the hoopla that surrounds the 14th to what surrounds the heart in the actual physiology of the human body. I believe oft times that heart disease is a gradual rejection of us by our heart of what we as a person still expect out of it, after years of mistreatment and bad habits.

If we expect our heart to perform well and feel good, we have to consistently guard it against unhealthy conditions or we will gradually experience a decline in performance, and eventually the chest pressure and the heart pains will begin and if not remedied, may lead to a heart attack, possibly causing permanent damage to parts of the heart or worse, death to the entire body.

Cardiovascular diseases kill way more people then any other illness that effects mankind, (it's the number one killer of Americans from all causes of death) and in addition tens of millions are significantly disabled by heart disease. Now that our government is the major medical care provider, cardiovascular diseases are costing American taxpayers hundreds of billions of dollars every year, so in that way even the healthy have to pay for other's bad habits that potentially lead to heart disease.

When we're not careful about the choices we make daily and the habits we form, a toxic environment will begin to grow in and around the heart causing the heart to not only begin to feel bad, but to also begin pumping toxins throughout the body until the whole body becomes sick. It may be a gradual process, but if we can go back in time and try to remember how things were when our heart was feeling good, strong and protected, we may be able to pick up on some good habits that got dropped along the way that will cause our heart to respond in a positive way.

Exercise, good deep rest and recovery, along with good heart healthy foods, time away from life's stresses for fun, relaxation and stress relief are great things that can show our heart that we care about everything it does for us and that we don't take it for granted! We may be able to take short cuts on these healthy habits for awhile, and sometimes it can take years before we realize the beginnings of heart disease, or even worse a heart attack where we either lose our life or at the least, life as we once knew it.

Our heart knows if we are doing things that only mask symptoms, so as to temporarily suppress reactions to mistreatment and negligence. If we don't get rid of these habits that started the problems in the first place, such as inactivity, bad diet, smoking, staying overstressed, using drinks that dehydrate instead of water to hydrate, and staying at a proper weight so as to not overburden our heart, it is comparable to giving a gift that appeals to the emotions of someone you care about on the 14th of February without following it up for the rest of the year with the things that helped make the relationship great in the first place!

It's probably no coincidence that the use of medicine has exploded in lockstep with packaged and processed food as has selfishness, divorce and stress with the explosion of heart disease over the past 30 years...

The basic, simple and wholesome things (such as clean air, clean water, healthy foods, exercise and deep rest), is what our heart responds to much more then the things that come in a box, bottle or a vial!

What we can do: at least 3-5 hours of medium to intense activity a week and try to break a sweat it helps your body get rid of toxins trapped inside! Get deep sleep, this is when our body recovers and gets back on top of things. Find a way to resolve the issues that are causing stress and get it out of your life and don't let it back in.

Note: the same hormone that stress produces also causes belly fat!

Diet: keep a regular water intake and keep heart healthy foods around so as to change habits without trying so hard. A diet rich in fruits, vegetables, nuts, eggs and other quality dairy products, fish, berries, healthy oils for the healthy fats along with beans and other foods rich in soluble fiber, these have cholesterol lowering benefits that statin drugs try to mimic.

When we do the above with consistency, it helps build the blood with good nutrients to build not only a strong heart, but a healthy environment around the heart leading to a strong cardiovascular system that will protect us from disease causing pathogens that want to invade and wreck the harmony of health that God has blessed us with.

AEROBIC EXERCISE VS. ANAEROBIC EXERCISE?

Over the past 20+ years of being in the health club business, I have seen many advancements made to exercise routines, supplements, exercise equipment, in-home exercise routines etc. Many fell by the wayside as fads that never gained traction in large part due to it not giving the rapid results they made people think they would get.

There are however some things that remain the same and give substance to why almost any exercise routine works:

1. Rapid continuous movement builds endurance and your aerobic/cardiovascular capacity

2. Putting your body under more strain then it's used to builds strength.

3. Eating a good diet and drinking plenty of water helps you with either of the above.

The Cardio vs. Strength training Myth:
throughout the years it has been common practice
to separate these two whether mentally or in actual
practice, but the lines are gradually blurring and
I'm really happy to see this. You see when 1 & 2 are
combined together you can build both in synch with
each other. You can build size and strength even if
you exercise slowly, but your endurance will not be
very good and I'm a firm believer that only after
endurance comes quality strength, tone or muscle
size. Think about it like this, if you get out in the
yard (whether at work or play) and you do
something rapidly and you tire easily, is it your
strength or cardio that needs strengthening, or is it
both? If you would do this same activity on a
regular basis, your body will fairly rapidly condition
itself to handle this new level of activity.

Example: if there is a hill that is fatiguing to you,
and you start walking it consistently and sometimes
rapidly, before long your regular pace will seem
very easy. Rapid movement through the same
distance builds muscle and (rapid movement
carried out for a longer session) will build strength

and endurance, exercise is as simple as that, it's cheap, its easy and the basics still work as good as they did in the caveman or hunter gatherer days.

Try this: get a set of dumbbells (whatever weight feels right for you) and do a deep squat touching them on the floor beside your ankles, keeping your back straight, then thrust back up raising them above your head, repeat until you get tired. Take 15 to 30 second breaks and repeat for at least 3-4 sets, (increase these sets according to your capability). You can gradually increase your speed or weight of your dumbbells to increase resistance. Remember to always warm up with a few sets that don't cause you to strain at first. If you can do these sets for about 10 minutes a day, you will begin to see results that far outweigh walking alone. The added muscle and tone not only looks much better then a shrunken shape, it also helps slow the aging process and speeds up metabolism!

1. Keep it simple and use movements that involve the larger muscle groups.

2. Do them more rapidly.

3. With less rest.

4. Gradually increase the load (added weight/resistance) we can have the benefits from both the aerobic/cardio and anaerobic/strength training!

 When a balanced approach is used, meaning muscle gains are equal to our cardiovascular conditioning, we have the benefit of strength that is matched with endurance, increased in bone strength, shaping up with the added muscle, along with the added metabolism benefit that comes with the extra muscle!

 When we make our muscles do a task faster it stimulates strength gain and if we do a task for a longer duration it stimulates the process that strengthens our cardiovascular system!

CONTROLLING SUGAR SPIKES...CONTROLS FAT DEPOSITS

Food intake is a lot like income, if we earn more then we spend, we have the opportunity to save some in case our income drops or is lost. Insulin is like our calorie banker, and once he or she satisfies the accounts that take care of our expenses, he or she puts the balance in our savings account (fat cells). This is our body's system working for us and we can't fault it for saving it if we're not giving it the toned muscle or the activity to burn the extra!

A lot of our food we consume does not have the recommended 5 grams of fiber per serving and we wind up eating much more then we should because we didn't get that full sensation in time. Much of our packaged foods have either added sugars or high fructose syrups (HFS) in them and this combination with starchy carbs is not something we want as part of our dietary intake if we're wanting to lose body fat or are trying to protect ourselves from diabetes. The one type of fiber (insoluble) helps make us feel full faster and the soluble fiber lines our digestive track with a sort of gel like substance and slows down the absorption of sugar into the bloodstream. The reason most fruits do not cause such a bad sugar spike as packaged or processed sweet food and beverages, is they contain the soluble fiber that helps regulate its absorption.

Our body produces insulin as a response to blood glucose (blood sugars) and delivers the energy from this glucose to working parts of the body to replenish their energy stores. Once this is completed and these cells have been replenished, it will start taking the leftover blood sugars to our fat cells, to store as reserve energy until our sugar runs low in our blood, the problem however is a lot of the foods we eat spike our blood sugar and do not allow this to happen. Our pancreas produces insulin in direct proportion to the amount of sugar in our blood at one time, so when a lot hits our bloodstream it produces a lot. This doesn't work well for keeping sugar levels steady because of the massive amount of insulin still in the blood looking for sugar! This is a lot of times when people repeat the cycle to get rid of that shaky feeling called a sugar low, instead of waiting a little while longer for the insulin levels to drop which will in turn trigger the release of energy stored in our fat cells or other wise known as burning fat.

There are a few things that will help avoid sugar spikes: skipping dessert after a high fat/high carb meal, eating half of a candy instead of the whole thing, no sweet drinks with meals, (however a sugared beverage that is consumed as part of a small snack when running on empty will mostly be sucked up by the body and used as energy), last but probably the most important, eat foods that take a while for your body to digest.

It's simple as this: insulin being in our blood locks up our fat cells and until our level of insulin drops down our body will not release energy from our fat cells. After insulin has done its job, it will start disappearing from our blood and this works as a trigger to release our other form of energy, (body fat).

Here are a few things we can do if we ate too much: inevitably this is going to raise our blood sugar levels and unless we get physically active after the meal, we are telling our insulin to do its job and store the excess in our fat cells. If we are active and our energy output is burning this extra off it doesn't have to store it because you have burned it. The times we really need to watch for are when we know we will be inactive; this is when these high-octane fuels can have a poisonous effect on our body.

When we eat too much lets do something Extra to burn off the Extra or the Extra is going to Extra size our fat cells!

SAFE FAT LOSS VS. TOXIC FAT LOSS

Almost every spring I see something that has repeated itself since I went into the health club business in 1991, and this is the desperate attempt at weight loss when we get close to spring and summer. This rapid weight loss can cause rapid aging and if you do it right, **there are a few things you can do that will ensure your efforts will yield the results you're after...**

1. Guard against muscle loss: oft times rapid weight loss results in a reduction in size and not so much the fat, (this is a lot of the reason our metabolism slows down). When we have a sudden drop in calories and we carry this new calorie schedule out long enough, our body will accommodate this by burning off however much muscle it needs to, to adjust to this low level of calories, this is what we know as slowing down our metabolism. This is simply our body's survival mechanism that works with us in famine conditions, so as to extend our life until we can find food. Remember our vital organs are made up of these highly metabolically active tissues as well and can lose their strength as well. This is how bad weight loss will result in aging a person, physical and organ strength drop off due to a loss of protein when your body slows your metabolism down during extended crash diets.

Our muscle (protein parts of the body) is highly metabolically active tissue and burns a lot of energy, so a large part of the health of our metabolism depends on our retention or our gain of muscle. When we build muscle and tone we build our body's capability of burning calories faster! And when we build muscle we gain good shape instead of the droop. This is what disappoints many with the results they see after rapid weight loss, when they see that 130 pounds (or whatever the goal weight was) simply don't look like it used to. Many younger people are very active and along with that activity comes muscle tone and when we try to lose weight without the activity, we have the weight loss without muscle tone.

2. Guard your body from fat cell toxicity: we come in contact with a lot of toxins whether environmental factors such as household cleaners, air refreshers, smoke along with toxins in our food supply, water and medications. When our body recognizes a toxin it protects the rest of the body from it with mucous or putting it in fat. When we lose weight rapidly without an antioxidant rich diet, plenty of water and plenty of sweat, we can have some very concentrated toxic leftovers in us. This can make us look sickly even though we're thin. These toxins can go on to create a rusting of sorts to our body parts that if not stopped can grow to a diagnosable and nameable disease. Eating plenty of fruits and vegetables throughout the weight loss period and beyond will help flush these toxins from your body along with plenty of sweat and water for elimination.

You were designed with natural mechanisms for weight loss, health and vibrancy that no man made fat burner, supplement or medication can match.

BREAKING THE FAST
AKA "Breakfast"

Break-fast comes from breaking the fast (going for about 7-10 hours of not eating during the night). There are many that extend this period out longer and do not break the fasting period until lunch or dinner, and this can be okay if it's not done every day, especially when we ate too much the evening or day before. This helps us burn off the excess fuel to keep our deposits to our fat cells in check.

You have probably experienced it or heard some- one say that when they eat cereal for breakfast that they seem to stay hungry. This comes from the insulin spike (from a breakfast made up primarily of simple carbs/sugars). This causes insulin to pour into our bloodstream for glucose distribution. The insulin transports the sugars off and continues to look for more, thus giving us a sugar low causing us to have intense sugar cravings. This is the fuel we have told our system it can expect for the day when we fed it this for breakfast. When we try to get it to shift over mid-day, we are apt to feel shaky until our body shifts over to a more steady form of energy, complex carbs, dietary fat and stored fat.

For Breakfast: I like to kick off the morning with some fruit; since this assists our body's natural detox processes. Other then this, I like a breakfast that largely consists of fat and protein, (this morning I had eggs poached in water, 1 slice of bread and 1/2 of a avocado). A breakfast primarily consisting of proteins and fats, gives you a steady fuel that will last and will help you avoid sugar spikes that lead to fat storage. If you want this benefit but want your diet to have a cholesterol lowering benefit, eat a little oatmeal or (drink a soluble fiber supplement such as BeneFiber) to force the body to pass the bile (bile breaks down fat) out through your waste, causing the liver to have to make new bile (our liver makes new replacement bile from cholesterol. This is the process that statin drugs try to mimic.

 If you eat or drink something sugary, avoid any caffeine as this causes a sugar trap in your blood due to temporary insulin insensitivity caused by the caffeine. I personally believe this is where a lot of our problems with blood fats/cholesterol, diabetes, and belly/organ fat are coming from.

We get to tell our body what energy it can expect by what we choose as starter fuel in the morning. It does not matter as much for someone that is going to be highly active after breakfast but VERY MUCH applies to someone that has a desk job or is going to be inactive over the next few hours. Sugar is torture to a body that has to set still!

A sugary or carb loaded breakfast is like high octane fuel that burns out rapidly and dies, while protein, fat and complex carbs are like logs that continue to emit a steady heat for hours!

SPORTS CONDITIONING VS. LIFESTYLE CONDITIONING

Sports conditioning is similar in concept to lifestyle specific conditioning, in that both are trying to maintain or, gain certain levels of capability. An athlete may lose his job if he is not conditioned properly, but anyone can lose the capability to live life the way they know it to be if they don't maintain their strength.

Exercising and the building of muscle and strength has many times gotten some scorn over the years and some of the contempt has probably been deserved because of the ones that take it to the extreme and get themselves looking like misshaped Tonka toys and seem to have no life beyond the gym and food…

Muscle conditioning and strengthening however is something that is applicable to everyone that wants to continue to do things for themselves, these are our activities of daily living (ADL's), and they can range from a very demanding physical job, to a person that has very limited physical mobility and are simply what each of us need to keep strong if we expect to continue being able to do these things on our own.

Strength and conditioning can be lifestyle specific whether its an athlete doing it for a particular sport, physical job, etc. and is simply what helps us get from A to Z in our individual respective days without so much of a struggle.

If we can keep in mind the (functional) movements we are doing now and the movements that we need to be able to do in the future, and then simply strengthen these movements, we can empower our lives by protecting and strengthening our capabilities for these activities and movements. This is applicable whether someone is a world-class soccer player all the way to someone that does not want to live their life out, stuck in a corner being dependent on others. The key is in making sure that our personal functional lifestyle movements stay strong.

Examples: if we walk up a hill every day, we can use this same hill to strengthen ourselves for a hiking trip or simply to strengthen these muscles, by carrying some hand weights along (anything that adds weight, such as two buckets filled to desired level with water). Since muscles adapt to new stresses, after doing this for a while, this will become easier and walking the hill without weights will become really easy. If we want to get up out of a squatting position easier, practice squatting and when it becomes easier, squat while holding some hand weights which will condition these particular muscles even further. If you get winded easily, simply do the things that cause you to get winded oftener and then do them faster and for longer periods! This will strengthen your heart and lungs along with your blood and oxygen delivery system. When your cardiopulmonary strength is built to match the rest of your physical strength, this = quality strength and conditioning.

Sports conditioning if done properly will push an athlete further then his or her prior conditioning level and this is why along with skill training he or she can be better when the next round of competition or sports season begins. This same thing applies to each of us in strengthening our weak points or gaining strength for future needs.

If we can keep in mind the movements we need now and the ones we need in our future and simply strengthen these functional lifestyle movements, our physical capabilities and our quality of life can become so much better and will give us what is called "A Good Economy of Movement."

Our body and its physiology was designed with adaptive capabilities to new stressors that mankind will never be able to duplicate, but is ours to enjoy and to deploy!

THE SKINNY ON SUMMER SHAPE-UP!

If you find yourself running out of winter and spring days to shape up for summer and are a part of the end of spring panic crowd, don't despair, its not too late if you don't use the wrong approach to shaping up or losing weight.

Have you ever noticed that two people can be the same height, frame, and weight with two complete different shapes? The reason is simple, the one has more muscle and the other has more fat. Oft times the one with more muscle is usually much more active, which will in turn burn more fat for energy, while toning, building and strengthening muscle which is where the added shape comes from.

Example: I took a member's body analyses when she started her exercise routine and she weighed in at 180. She was very serious and stuck with her routine over the next 2 months and she really shaped up, looked very healthy and had a younger look about herself. BUT she had gained 2 pounds and was at 182. When we took the analysis again we were able to see why she looked so different at about the same weight, she had dropped 20 pounds of fat weight and gained 22 pounds of lean weight giving her a complete different look!

When you begin a fitness routine, you want to give yourself at least 2 months of muscle conditioning time before expecting to see a lot of weight loss on the scale. Throughout our life as we mature, we gain muscle, and any good conditioning program will help you regain this former muscle tone, bringing with it, renewed metabolism and bone density!

Rather then have such a bend toward how thin we can be by a certain date, we should aim toward seeing how toned we can get the underlying muscle which will firm things up even if at a larger size and will look much healthier and shapely then a thin untoned shape. Lots of times a side effect of rapid weight loss is a saggy appearance and a sickly look can come from the rapid release of toxic substances from fat cells into our system.

Fast Routine: do a full body routine (minimum of 3 rounds) that involves squatting movements for the lower body along with exercises that involve the pulling and pushing muscles of the upper body (different angles helps force different muscles to work harder). These exercises can be bench-presses or pushups, bent rows, and squats. For stomach, low back and core do leg raises, crunches and planks.

Going directly from one muscle group to the next, is key to keeping the heart rate up and your lungs working to produce more oxygen into the blood, (this will help you get cardiovascular conditioning and stimulates the release of body fat for energy along with the added muscle tone). Speed of exercise movement also helps muscle to tone more rapidly.

Weight we all need to lose: depending on the types of foods we eat and our age, we can be holding up to 20+ pounds of residue/waste in our midsection. Removing this sludge is important, not only for a flat belly area, but for our health as well. Eating mostly raw fruits, vegetables, nuts, and beans for about 5-7 days can be a real belly flattener, (due to the removal of excess intestinal waste). Add in some oils to your salads and vegetables to help with the cleanse (fish oil caps can help as well). Drinking a warm cup of water with the juice from 1 squeezed lemon, (add lemon juice after heating the water), can really help the detoxifying process in the morning and boost your immune system!

Our approach to weight loss and fitness can have an aging and sagging effect or a toning, firming and rejuvenating effect! Our body and its systems have to last us for the rest of our life and it's worth doing it right!

UNLEASHING YOUR INNER PHARMACY! 6 BEST DOCTORS

When foreign invaders come into our body and attempt to upset the balance, it would make any of us feel good if we could see the armies unleashed by our immune system. It not only fights it back, but just like an evolving, ever learning computer system, it will archive the new data it has learned throughout generations of immune cells and once it knows the sequence of these pathogens, (our innate immune system) will destroy them many times without us realizing we made contact with something bad. Our immune system is adaptive and just like our muscles and bones, when exposed to new stressors, and given the proper amount of recovery after the new stressor, will become stronger.

Our inner pharmacy knows the designer medicine it needs to release to kill these pathogens, but just like any manufacturing and production facility, it has a few things that it needs from us. This is a checklist I like to hand out to everyone and is something I feel we all need to check ourselves against before unnecessarily worrying a doctor or taking things created in a laboratory that can oft times create another problem while attempting to correct the current one.

1. Am I getting fresh air? We die most rapidly without the ingredient it contains, (oxygen)! Don't breath in bad things especially not on purpose...

2. Am I drinking 1/2 of my bodyweight in ounces of water? We are made up of several trillion cells and can die within 3 days without hydration, so in a very short amount of time we can dry out and kill several billion cells, causing things to hurt and fatigue!

3. Have I been eating healthy foods? We are what we eat, look closely at it and then ask a simple question, do I want cells to be made of this? Your body likes foods that contain only one ingredient. The more ingredients it has, the more its processed and the further it is from natural and the less your body recognizes it as good nutrition.

4. Have I been staying active, or getting exercise? Our body and its functions work better physiologically if we move our body parts and when these hold still for too long circulation suffers in the short term and weakening of muscle, tendons ligaments and bones in the long term, causing us to lose our good economy of movement as we age.

5. Am I staying at the proper weight? Just like a vehicle that is loaded down with a lot of extra weight for long enough, will begin to experience wear and tear on small minor parts and eventually if not relieved of its load will prematurely age the vital part. The difference is that our human body parts are not so easily replaced or replicated.

6. Am I getting adequate rest? If you're not getting deep rest, figure out why not, it is that important! This is when your body repairs things and gradually you will not only feel run down, your body's defenses will lose their armor and can be much easier for bad things (pathogens) to breach and make you sick.

7. Am I getting plenty of sunshine? Your immune system doesn't care about that certain tanned look that many want only certain times out of the year, what it cares about is that it helps restore vitamin d levels naturally. After scaring people into believing the sun is bad for us (something that's been around since God created the world and is important to life), they have linked all sorts of illness and disease to Vitamin D deficiency! Length of exposure should be gradual and based on skin type.

When we do the above consistently, it empowers a system that is like a personal doctor at work within us 24 x 7 x 365 days a year that knows exactly what is wrong and what to do to fix it!

WATER RETENTION

Most of us have probably had this come up either personally or with someone we know. Water retention is something that if we can bring into balance, (when we are retaining water) can yield some pretty rapid weight loss, but when done in a forced unhealthy manner, will not look good and certainly will not be healthy, since there is an underlying reason behind this retention of fluid and is something that should be addressed to keep us from continuing to pit laboratory designed chemicals against our body's natural regulatory hormonal and chemical processes.

There are a few main things we should look at to help keep things in balance naturally and some of the main ones are...

1. Staying hydrated.

2. Keeping our sodium and potassium in balance.

Staying hydrated: when we let our selves dehydrate it sets off survival mechanisms to protect our fluid levels and will do this by concentrating the urine (it will be a lot darker) and it does this to conserve fluid for the blood plasma and other cellular activity.

Our pituitary gland monitors our plasma levels in our blood and if it seems to be getting low during periods of dehydration (oft times our blood pressure will also be low) it will then trigger the release of arginine vasopressin (an antidiuretic hormone) into the blood causing the adrenals (which set on top of the kidneys) to release aldosterone.

The above processes trigger the kidneys into reabsorbing fluids that were going to be urine and simply concentrating it down so that as little fluid as possible is lost through the urine. This also encourages the reabsorption of sodium for the purpose of the body being able to retain more fluids so that this dehydration that just happened will not happen again. Once a person has hydrated for long enough, and the arginine vasopressin levels start dropping, the exact opposite happens and sodium starts getting released along with the extra fluid retention. I like to think of this as; once our body is thoroughly convinced that we are not in a drought situation it will stop retaining extra water and will release it according to the level of satisfaction reached. Alcohol is a very bad diuretic and if someone binge drinks it can lead to at least several days of fluid retention and can last longer if a person does not properly hydrate.

 We react no differently as an individual when we store up for uncertain times ahead, this is oft times in direct proportion to the level of hardship a person went through or has seen in their life and can turn some people into real pack rats, our body's subconscious survival mechanisms work exactly the same.

 Sodium and Potassium balance: I like to think of sodium as something that draws in and

potassium as something that releases. It's like a

room that keeps letting people through the entrance without a properly working exit door it can get uncomfortably full of people. We need both sodium and potassium in balance to allow hydration, but when we continue to consume piles of salt with low intake of potassium, our body will continue to hydrate until we see what we recognize as fluid retention.

There has been many clinical trials done that shows increasing our potassium intake and decreasing our sodium intake can reduce blood pressure, leading to a reduced risk of heart attack, heart failure, stroke and according to 3 new studies would prevent millions of deaths per year from heart disease and stroke!

We need to reduce our sodium intake down to 3-4 grams a day and increase our potassium intake along with at least 1/2 our body weight in ounces of water.

Some foods rich in potassium are: bananas, apricots, cantaloupe, honeydew, oranges, grapefruit, tomatoes, prunes, green leafy vegetables, root vegetables, seeds, legumes, potatoes, lima beans, almonds, sunflower seeds and molasses.

Urine monitoring: we should try to keep our urine a pale yellow. Darker yellow means we're not drinking enough water, and completely clear may mean we're drinking too much. Drinking too much water can cause us to wash too many minerals out, which in turn can lead to fluid imbalance.

Our body not only has a well designed immune system, but also an equally well designed system of survival that will retain water according to the level of drought we subjected it to.

A.G.E.'s AND AGING

Something that I've been following for a while now, is a process (that can happen to food before consumption and in our body after consumption of sugary foods, especially the ones with fructose), that is a large contributing factor in premature aging and many of the diseases associated with aging such as: skin disorders, cancer, heart disease, type II diabetes, kidney disorders, atherosclerosis, high blood pressure, Alzheimer's, stroke and visual impairment. This is a process called Advanced Glycation End Products (AGE's), that we can simply interpret as a dangerous end product of food prepared wrong and too much of a sugar load in the body). There are two main causes of these advanced glycation end products...

Through our food preparation: this happens when we brown our foods and usually is the result of protein and sugars binding together through things such as a grilling, frying or baking process. It may give added taste and appearance, but it has a nasty effect on food value. An example of this is the top of a loaf of bread after baking and other pastries such as cookies, doughnuts etc. Basically these Advanced Glycation End Products (AGE's) happen when heating or cooking sugars with proteins in the absence of water. These sugar and protein molecules that bond together in a hard crusty like fashion is sort of what happens on the walls of our veins and arteries as well. Fructose undergoes this glycation process at about 10 times the rate as glucose and most sweeteners are around 50% fructose or a fructose derivative, (this is bad stuff and can be found in most processed foods).

The 2nd way these AGE's are formed is in our body: sugars that are not burned off as energy can bind to proteins as well. When this happens, it can alter not only the structure, but the function of the protein as well.

Example: collagen is made up of protein and is found all throughout the body in skin, muscle, organs, veins and arteries and gives elasticity and cohesion to these structures. When sugar product binds to these proteins it not only changes the way it is shaped but also how it functions. This causes that particular part of us to have premature aging, such as our skin losing its elasticity, muscle shrinkage and weakness, veins and arteries (not being able to dilate or constrict properly), heart disease, brain disease, the beginnings of a cancer cluster, or a pancreas that is just plain sick of all the sugar load and decides it can no longer produce adequate insulin to remove all these sugars from the blood.

Glucose and protein are meant to work together for energy but when there is to much sugar, it is way too much sticky matter throughout our system and when it bonds with these protein structures it wreaks havoc and makes things get older a lot faster and in some cases we don't age evenly and develop a bad batch of cells that get diagnosed as one of the chronic diseases.

Simple things we can do: avoid processed food and drinks, especially the sugary ones and try to fill in with more raw fruits, vegetables and nut snacks, drink half your body weight in ounces of water, (you'll be surprised what you will crowd out of your food and drink schedule simply by adding these in). Try to prepare foods in a way that don't cause them to lose their color, cook and grill meats etc. at lower temperatures, dark chocolate for that sweet tooth, avoid caffeine with sugary combinations and last but not least, don't trust food and drink items with multiple ingredients in them, especially not the ones that have ingredients you don't recognize, chances are your body will not either, and foods like these are the ones that cause advanced glycation end products that in turn cause premature aging and disease. Exercise/activity is something that can help burn off these excess sugars.

Mixing in enough healthy habits to dilute down the bad habits can help our body in lengthening out our health span to closer match our lifespan, with the end goal being a match!

THE IMPORTANCE OF FIBER

Fiber can be one of your best friends when it comes to weight loss and slenderizing the mid-section, but there is a lot more that can be appreciated about fiber beyond it's cosmetic effects, such as a cancer reduction risk and many more benefits. The National Cancer Institute found a 22% reduction in cancer if men consumed 30 grams per day and women 25 grams per day.

I like to think of fiber content as a good judge of a food's character, if the content is too low, (less then 5 grams per serving) the consumer should be aware of potential side effects! This is primarily for the carbohydrate group of foods and not so much for the protein and fat groups. However even with the protein and fat groups, we should be sure to include plenty of fiber for the purpose of helping move this otherwise waxy glob through our digestive track and to help control our cholesterol. Carbs without fiber is almost like consuming pure sugar and this helps cause diabetes and rapid weight gain.

There are a few important things to understand about fiber and how the two types work that will help us become better judges of our foods. It helped me understand better how the two worked when I knew a primary difference between the two, soluble fiber will dissolve in water and insoluble fiber will not.

The soluble fiber turns into a sort of gel substance and puts a slight film through our digestive track which slows the absorption of nutrients down, which in turn keeps the flow of nutrients more steady when entering the bloodstream and avoids those spikes and crashes. Soluble fiber is the reason we can eat most fruits without worrying about a sugar spike like we do when we eat or drink processed sweets such as, sodas, fruit drinks, sweet tea, candies and deserts, this is also the reason foods rich in soluble fiber are so important to diabetics and ones wanting to avoid diabetes.

Soluble fiber also has a cholesterol lowering effect!

The process: we excrete bile from our gall bladder when we eat foods containing fat and this bile helps our digestive track break down these fats.

Normally this bile gets reabsorbed and used again, but if we can keep the bile from reabsorbing, it causes the liver to have to make new bile salts, and our liver makes this bile from cholesterol. So eating foods that have a high content of soluble fiber can be your natural cholesterol lowering statin.

The insoluble fiber adds bulk to our foods which helps us realize that we have eaten enough, which in turn avoids that realization about 20 minutes after consumption that we have eaten and drank about 500 calories too many. It also helps break up otherwise big globules of food that can slide into and stick in crevices of our digestive track. This insoluble fiber helps massage this old and new food up out of these curves and crevices, helping provide us with a clean digestive track. When our body is absorbing nutrients from our digestive track instead of toxins (from years of built up residue leaching back into our system) we will see energy levels improve and our defense against chronic disease!

Note: if you eat prior to a period of inactivity, this is an especially important time to only eat foods that have plenty of fiber. Liquid sugar drinks (including fruit juices, sports drinks etc.) are a disaster to attempts at weight loss and are extremely bad for sugar spikes and crashes. Try to have 5 grams of fiber per serving.

Information exercise: do an Internet search by entering "Foods rich in soluble fiber" and "Foods rich in insoluble fiber," copy down these foods on separate lists, then surround yourself with the ones you like on these individual lists and you will be surprised how easy it is to get your daily fiber needs.

Soluble fiber helps us control sugar spikes and cholesterol, insoluble fiber is our food mover and the cleaner of our digestive track!

RESEARCHING FOR LIFESTYLE OFFSETS

Oft times there is a lifestyle change or changes we can find to help counter health problems or even genetic weaknesses that gives us future health concerns. It's like boarding up and reinforcing a window that is facing an upcoming storm that could potentially slam foreign objects into the house's weak spot.

Example: if there is weakness or pain in your hip, use a cane (this should speed up the healing process or at the least prevent further injury).

The first thing we need to is a diagnosis of our weakness, whether a present condition or one we have a genetic weakness for due to family health history, and depending what the condition is, (we may need a medical specialist to help put a pinpoint on the condition). Once we have this, whether through personal diagnosis, or medical assistance, we should become proactive with our diet and other lifestyle choices that strengthen our weakness. This can be for most chronic and physical conditions. This approach is all about lifestyle offsets!

Most of us probably have some concerns about our future access to healthcare and what limitations will be put on certain procedures and medications. I personally feel that so much access to healthcare throughout the years has made us less proactive in taking responsibility in the things that keep our body healthy, such as avoiding obesity, eating healthy foods instead of processed foods, drinking water instead of caffeinated-carbonated-syrup drinks, breathing clean air and avoiding breathing pollutants into our lungs and blood supply such as cigarette smoke and the list goes on. And the way the healthcare bill seems to be shaping up this dependence will lead to an uncertain reliance.

Here are a few steps we can take to counter our ailments and weaknesses:

1. Understand what the problem is. This may require medical diagnosis, but there is a lot of research someone can do online for free. Online research can yield a lot if you can describe what it is you want information on. The better your

description, the better the search results. It's a lot

the same with the doctor, if you don't describe your symptoms clearly; it makes it a lot harder for him or her to diagnose the problem.

2. Where it is coming from? This is where we figure out what it is that is causing the problem and where the problem or symptom is getting its energy. If we can find and squash this, problem solved!

3. What lifestyle changes we can apply to this condition? Many times there are things we can correct in our diet or other lifestyle habits that can give our body the tools it needs to correct the problem(s).

Example: if we have type 2 diabetes or have symptoms of it and want to get our diet on track to do our proactive counter attack, simply do a search

like this: "best diet for diabetes." I like typing in

"livestrong" behind most of my research questions; it's a really great free resource.

4. Apply these changes! This is one of the most important steps we can take to start turning things around!

5. Consistency! Consistency is the key to effectiveness and very important if we want our efforts from all the above to have effect!

6. Patience! Doing it naturally may seem to take longer, (some medications are very necessary) but when done naturally our body does it without a smorgasbord of side effects that our body has to recover from, when we take unnecessary medications.

When we do these above listed steps, we are giving our body the tools it needs to fix problems and or to strengthen against genetical weaknesses.

Example information exercise: type into your Internet search bar; "best exercises for lowering blood pressure." Select the link that you like best, read that article and then looks on the right side of the page and you will find a list of links that will help you narrow your research. This can apply to questions on weight loss, chronic disease, bone and joint problems, exercise questions etc.

When we focus like a laser on something for 30+ minutes we can gain knowledge about the issue we're worried about and since knowledge = power, the more knowledge you gain, the more leverage you have against the problem. The remaining step is application!

You cannot expect your doctor to care as much as you do about your own condition. When we know and understand a problem, the less likely we are to accept it as an ongoing condition.

THE DESIGNER COLORS
OF NUTRITION

This is one of my favorite subjects, especially this time of year when locally grown produce starts becoming available! We have shaped a food industry that largely caters to fast and packaged food markets, due to the demand we as consumers have placed on these food like products and it's

showing up in not only the obesity epidemic but also the ensuing onslaught of chronic disease in this country!

All the different colors a variety of fruits and vegetables provide are different nutrients and they serve different purposes in the body.

Examples: green color, helps our vision, orange color helps vision, healthy skin and our immune system, red color helps improve heart health and lowers risk of cancer, purple color reduces cancer risk, anti-aging, and supports mental clarity, white color (as in onions) helps reduce cholesterol levels, lowers blood pressure and helps prevent diabetes. Getting a variety of colors throughout a 7-10 day period is important to insure that these nutrients stay at protective levels in our blood. This is what helps build our immunity to potentially harmful things whether by contact or consumption.

What really turns these vegetables and fruits into designer packets of nutrition is if it is locally grown and consumed. I strongly believe the things that grow in an area help people deal with environmental conditions of that area and that they are a part of our body's checks and balances and the more we eat from outside sources the more imbalanced our inner health will become, (sort of like thinking the same set of tires that works on a car in the south will work on a car that faces icy conditions in the north). In other words nature has a reason that the Noni berry grows well in the South Pacific, the orange grows really well in Florida and the peach grows really well in Georgia, they are nature's packets of multi vitamin and minerals designed by that area for that area. Another example is how honeybees use local pollen for production of honey produced in and area and this same honey will sort of vaccinate you against allergy problems because it's made from the pollen in this same area.

We don't need a lot of space to grow a small garden and probably most of us have an area of our yard that could be a lot more productive then growing grass! We can also support and purchase more of our fruits and vegetables from the roadside stands and farmers markets in our area, these are the ones that bridge the gap between farmer and consumer in our local areas!

If we can start as an individual, family, community, and county, to change what we perceive as good food and change what we consume, we can change the status of health and fitness in our region!

By becoming a community that lives and breathes health and fitness, we can empower the internal systems God blessed us with and decrease our need for medicine and medical interventions!

Support your local Farmacies aka produce stands; they are our natural source for localized multivitamins, immunization, and medications that help condition us against what we face locally!

MY FUN IN THE SUN, IS IT DANGEROUS?

Have you ever wondered why people seem so healthy during the summer? It very likely comes from more time spent outside and in the sun, where our body can naturally produce nature's only hormonal vitamin...vitamin D!

When we change the way nature is set up (for us) to be participants of, we need to keep in mind that nature can be a little environmentally harsh to someone who is not conditioned to it at all when they suddenly over expose themselves to these environmental conditions! Even a overexposure to a health club could be bad for our muscles, tendons, ligaments and joints, it's no different with the sun on our skin!

We need professionals that advocate gradual conditioning of the skin rather then promoting the daily slathering on of chemicals and in so many words saying we should trust chemicals more then something that has been around for 1000's of years (the sun) and something the human body is designed to naturally protect itself from through the production of a hormonal vitamin!

 Warning against over exposure is a good thing, but professionals making claims that the sun is bad for people, is one of the most ignorant ones I've ever heard! These claims probably somehow stem from the multi billion dollar skin care industry.

 Research studies and claims always make me curious when they come up with negative results on things that have been a part of people's lives for thousands of years. A curious thing happened after the media and other sources scared many people into protecting themselves against the sun's deadly rays, (chronic disease sky rocketed)! And most of these chronic diseases are associated with low vitamin D levels! Research published in the Archives of Internal Medicine shows that those with the lowest levels of vitamin D have more than double the risk of dying over an eight-year period and they cited the reason for these deficiencies was decreased outdoor activity. When I looked up vitamin D and chronic disease, there were 16,300,000 results! One thing the naysayers cannot dispute, is that all life here on earth would cease to function without the sun.

One of vitamin D's many processes in the body: when we produce adequate levels of vitamin D, it helps us pull calcium from the foods we eat that contain calcium. When our vitamin D levels are low our calcium levels in the body drop even if we have a calcium rich diet, this in turn will force the body to pull calcium from the bones for muscle activity etc. thus making our bones brittle and weak!

A cascading effect of vitamin D: low levels of vitamin D will cause low levels of calcium, low levels of calcium will cause our body to be less alkaline. This means our body becomes more acidic and a body that is more acidic becomes more disease friendly! I believe these acidity levels have contributed in a major way to the epidemic of chronic disease we have now.

Here's a little trick to get around buying vitamin D made in a laboratory: Spend 5-20 minutes in the mid-day sun with as much skin exposed as possible, (exposure time should vary by fairness of skin). Experts say 10 minutes will give your body enough radiation to manufacture about 10,000 IU of vitamin D. The neat thing is that our body can store extra vitamin D in our fat cells for the winter (vitamin D is fat soluble), so I think its pretty easy to see what God gave us summers for! The further north you live, the more you may benefit from additional vitamin D supplementation.

Quick notes: there are 3 types of ultraviolet rays A, B, & C. UVA rays are the most common and reach beyond the top layer of skin, UVB is mostly absorbed by the ozone layer but some makes it through especially at mid-day and is responsible for the production of vitamin D, UVC is the dangerous kind and is mostly absorbed by the ozone layer.

Tanning beds: produce both A & B rays but primarily A.

Note: the key to healthy sun therapy is in gradual exposure and avoiding long periods of overexposure after long periods of underexposure. Remember that (just like our muscle, bones, immune system as well as other physiological functions in our body), our skin is not so different in that it becomes conditioned for a gradual increased exposure to a particular condition, and when we overdo something, things break down and when we continue to do this it can lead to a chronic inflammatory condition which is the root of most chronic disease!

Foods good for skin color: some foods that are really good for healthy skin color are dark-orange foods which are loaded with vitamin A such as: cantaloupe, sweet potatoes, apricots, orange and yellow peppers.

Skin protection: colorful compounds (carotenoids) from fruits and vegetables get deposited in the skin and protect against sunburn and oxidation aka aging of the skin.

Remember to build exposure gradually and just like a muscle steadily becomes stronger and avoids injury with gradual resistance your skin will also build its protection and produce an awesome supply of natural vitamin D the way you were designed to receive it. I hope you have a lot of fun in the sun this summer and get plenty of vitamin D stored up for fall and winter!

A FAT BURNING ENVIRONMENT

Our calorie sources, activities and environment that we keep ourselves surrounded with will not only shape us mentally and physically but will also shape our future health as well.

I will try to address these three separately so that you can pin point weak spots that may be causing sticking points in your weight loss goals, (however, when these three are combined, you have a fat burning tool chest)!

1. Our Calorie Sources: the choices we make for our calorie's dictates to the body our intention for our energy needs. This is why, when we eat or drink something that absorbs rapidly, it puts a lot of glucose/sugar in our blood for energy. If this energy is not needed due to inactivity, our body will store this extra energy in our fat cells causing them to get bigger. And since our body burns off sugars first, it will not release stored fat into our blood to burn until our sugar is low enough to switch energy sources.

When we eat excess calories, especially the fast absorbing ones and we don't burn this extra off through exercise or activity, our insulin if working properly will remove it from our blood to keep from a sticky mess happening in our blood supply and our body parts!

The neat thing about our body is that it knows how to release an energy snack into our system when we need it badly enough and it does this by releasing the calories we have stored in our fat cells, body fat is simply stored energy.

Remember when eating lean or very low calorie for several days you should have a cheat meal, (where you eat and drink pretty much anything you want). This cheat meal simply helps reset your metabolism at a higher level.

2. Activities & Exercise: this is really important since activities and exercise not only burn calories while being active, but also help you continue to burn calories through the toned muscles these activities and exercises help create. The more toned muscle you have the higher your metabolism will be. One pound of muscle will burn approximately 13-17 calories a day. Activating these muscles will change it to a higher calorie burn rate, sort of like a car that burns fuel if left idling but will burn even more when revved up or in motion.

Simply put, activity and exercise help clear the system of excess energy so insulin will not have to tote it off to store in our fat cells for later.

3. Our Environment: getting family, friends and co-workers to support our fitness lifestyle can be of big benefit not only to us, but it can have a ripple effect on the ones around us! We gradually become like our environment, so it's very important to keep things and people around that have a positive impact and not a negative one on our fitness goals!

Calorie Sources: surround yourself (kitchen and workplace) with foods such as fish, chicken breasts, turkey, occasional good quality red meats, eggs, beans, dark colored vegetables, sweet potato, quinoa, brown rice, whole grain pasta, fermented vegetables and snacks such as apples, nuts, peanut butter (without the bread). Drink 1/2 your body weight in oz. of water. **Note:** cold water helps your body burn more calories.

When you combine a cleaned up fitness environment, active lifestyle, and good dietary choices with water as a fluid of choice you have a fat burning tool chest that helps turn that stored energy (body fat) into a burnable fuel!

WATER IS A FREE FAT BURNER!

Water's effect on the metabolism has been something that has intrigued me for years! The reason we do not hear more about it is simple, supplement companies and pharmaceutical companies do not sell water, they sell fat burners and metabolism boosters in pill form and try to duplicate natural processes in a resell-able form.

Foods we consume are measured by calories and when we eat extra calories beyond the fuel we need for energy, our body will simply store these for later use in our fat cells. Calories are simply units of heat/energy and are relied on for energy in our body whether its for our daily activities, digestion or temperature control. There are certain things that have a thermogenic effect in our body that will cause the body to release this stored energy (body fat) as usable heat/energy.

Water has ZERO calories, but the body has to expend units of heat (calories) to warm up this water, which can lead to a thermogenic (fat releasing) effect on our fat cells causing them to release energy.

A large portion of our required daily calories are used for controlling temperature, whether it's to cool us, or to heat us and our body will work hard to keep our thermostat ay 98.6 degrees.

Example: according to the American Counsel on exercise, you can burn up to 400 calories an hour from shivering. The way I would interpret this, is if there are not enough calories from food in the digestive system, this shivering is causing a thermogenic (fat burning) process, causing a release of energy from our fat cells for heating purposes.

A similar process happens for the sweating process when the body is pumping water through our cooling system and this is what keeps us from overheating. Our body when given enough water during times of heat, is really good at pushing this heat out and it burns lots of calories keeping our temperature where its supposed to be!

Each pound of fat holds approximately 3,500 calories, and when these units of energy are released whether for heating the body, cooling the body or for daily activities and exercise, it works like the energy we get from food except is has the slenderizing effect many of us our looking for.

A study that was published in the Journal of Clinical Endocrinology and Metabolism showed that drinking about 2 cups of water increases metabolism by 24%. That sounds like a lot to me and I don't know exactly how the groundwork was laid to arrive at this percentage, but when you figure that every single action and reaction in the body is reliant on hydration, this could be a very reasonable increase.

When we imagine our several trillion cells needing hydration, there has got to be a lot of activity when water enters the body and gets transported throughout our system.

Which is best, cold or room temperature? Water has been shown to increase the metabolism even when water was 98.6 (normal body temperature), and I believe its because of the simple fact that our body kicks into overdrive whenever we give it the product it needs to hydrate the several trillion cells in our body and it takes this job very seriously since hydration is next in line to oxygen, when it comes to survival!

However if you want to increase the thermogenic (fat burning) effect it has on the body, drink it cold. Your body has to burn calories (units of heat) to get cold water's temperature up to body temperature at 98.6 degrees, so the colder the water the more calories (units of heat) our body has to burn to get it to body temperature.

If we knew how good clean water tastes (with no additives, chemicals, or sugar) to the trillions of cells in our body, it would taste like dessert to our mouth!

INSULIN SPIKES AND FATTY DEPOSITS

I was watching a health segment about diabetes on a local news channel and the approach to the subject matter seemed really weird. They were discussing diabetes and were targeting red meat and saturated fats as the primary culprit. I never once heard them warn against a carbohydrate loaded diet, sugars, caffeine/sugar combinations, or high fat meals with sugary/starchy sides, which are the real culprits and enemies of the pancreas (our insulin source).

I'm not an advocate however, of a lot of red meat in the diet, since most of what's available is not from range fed beef sources and it is not as easily digested as other sources of protein, such as fish, nuts, beans and lentils.

Studies like this that go up against things that have been in our diets as long as people have been on earth usually don't bother addressing the substantiating factors that shape their research, such as loads of condiments, white bread, fries, sugared drinks and desserts instead of vegetables, beans, lentils and other things that are loaded with soluble fiber, (the ingredient that helps control sugar and cholesterol when consuming fats and carbs).

Research like this is like someone placing nails in the pathway of tires and then claiming that the rubber is bad because of all the cases of flat tires coming into the tire shops.

The way insulin works: our body releases insulin in response to our sugar rising above fasting blood sugar levels. Our insulin has got to deposit it somewhere, because if it don't and a lot of sugar stays in the blood it will kill us graveyard dead! Most cases of diabetes have to do with over taxation of the pancreas with loads of sugar and foods that break down rapidly into sugar.

The cells of our body really appreciate insulin helping them get adequate sugar/glucose for energy, but they don't appreciate it when insulin is continuing to try to get them to take in something they already have enough of and they will then start to form a resistance to the insulin, forcing the pancreas to produce more insulin which will force the cells to uptake more energy causing them to swell and get fat. This would be like a parent forcing a child to do something over and over that is not good for him or her, which will result in this child growing up resisting the parent, perhaps to the extent that communication is dead by the time he or she is older, creating a need for outside intervention.

Constant acute insulin spikes and levels cause: insulin insensitivity and it overworks our pancreas, eventually causing a person to depend on medicine to keep insulin levels steady.

When we eat high fat foods with high carb/sugar combinations, it creates a perfect storm for fatty deposits, insulin will flood our system to keep blood sugar levels in check and insulin will then not only increases the storage of fat in fat cells but will also prevent the release of fat as burnable energy!

There are 8 hormones that stimulate fat burning: epinephrine, norepinephrine, adrenocorticotrophic hormone, glucagon, thyroid-stimulating hormone, melanocyte-stimulating hormone, vasopressin and growth hormone.

There is ONE hormone that prevents the release of fat as energy: insulin.

 What we can do:

1. Avoid eating/drinking sugars and fast digesting carbohydrates with meals that are high in fat. Avoid packaged snacks that have less then 5 grams of fiber per 25 grams of carbs.

2. If you mess up and overdo it, exercise or get active for the next hour or so (after a meal) doing something that requires physical activity, this will help burn off these blood sugars and take the burden off the pancreas by making our muscle cells hungry for energy, thus making them more receptive to glucose delivery from insulin that is attempting to lower blood sugar to safe levels.

3. Add in cinnamon or cinnamon capsules with your meals. Cinnamon has an antioxidant that makes our cells more sensitive to insulin, which means our pancreas doesn't have to work as hard.

In summary: it's what we eat with what we eat and coincidentally the same thing (diet and exercise) helps most of us avoid diabetes or get rid of it. Doing this also helps us turn on our fat burning switch!

HOW MY DNA CAN MAKE ME LOOK OLDER OR YOUNGER

Our DNA (inside our cells) holds the blue print for how we look in the future, and it's largely up to us whether it's a gradual or rapid appearance of aging.

Part of the reason this is so intriguing to me is that we can strengthen the blueprint through common healthy habits done with consistency. Our DNA is inside each of our cells just like a memory bank or computer that holds a copy of instructions on how to continue to build replicas of itself.

When we think of the fact that our body is made up of several trillion cells and that these cells have DNA inside each of them that instructs how the next cell generation is made, it becomes more important to us, to not do things to our body that mess up these instructions, which pretty much happens every year to build the several trillion new generation of cells! This is involves, bone cells, heart cells, lung cells, skin cells, and all the cells that give the elasticity and shape to our body!

Bad habits to our body are a lot like a bad environment in a kitchen where a recipe is exposed to the these conditions and though the recipe gets hard to read, you still have to prepare the recipe the best you can, very likely the outcome will not taste or look like it was originally supposed to.

When we breathe in smoke and other pollutants instead of clean oxygen, drink fluids filled with processed sugars, phosphoric acid and caffeine, instead of good clean water, eat processed foods made inside a plant instead of from a plant, get caffeinated instead of rest and rejuvenation and then top it off by staying out of the sun like as if we're vampires and think it better to take laboratory produced vitamin D; we give our DNA no choice but to build a more sickly generation of cells, causing what we see as premature aging or diagnosed as one of the chronic diseases.

Taking vitamin D supplementation in my opinion is good, but taking it to completely replace the sun and your natural production of vitamin D is not.

Good habits on the other hand will not only protect the DNA, but will also fuel the DNA with good nutrients to produce a healthier generation of replicas, helping avoid the appearance of rapid aging.

The neat thing is that even a person that has had years of bad habits can start turning this around by practicing basic healthy habits, this is why someone can look years younger then they used to years earlier.

Diet: keeping plenty of fruits and vegetables in our diet will help us get the daily antioxidants to get rid of the oxidation that otherwise will build up in our body. Oxidation is what causes rusting on a scratched vehicle and will have a similar effect on our cells causing our DNA to give out mixed signals on how to build the next generation of cells, causing our appearance to begin to change.

Water, Exercise and Sweat, helps our body push out the toxins that build up in our body assisting our body's elimination process. When our body only gets to eliminate these toxins through urination and feces, the chances go up that they will build up in our body causing premature aging and degenerative disease.

Our body was created by a Creator that designed it to fight aging and degenerative disease, and it only asks for some basic tools to do its job…

These primary tools are:

1. Clean Air.

2. Clean Water.

3. Healthy Balanced Diet.

4. Activities and Exercise.

5. Sunshine.

6. Things that Challenge the Brain.

7. Good deep rest.

Good habits are to our several trillion cells like a recipe that is on a laminated page that is protected against a tough kitchen environment. The chances that this particular recipe will give clear easy to read instructions years later is much better.

BINGE MEALS AND BURNING FAT

A binge meal is the one thing besides the goal of burning fat that is looked forward to in most calorie restricting diets. The nice thing is that we can do this and actually assist our body in the fat burning process by having these occasional cheat meals.

Over the years I have had a lot of people that were on strict diets, tell me that it seemed that when they binged out a little, that it seemed to spark their weight loss, there is a good reason for this and the scale was not being deceptive to them.

Our body works in a really neat way in detecting when we are not getting as many calories as we need and when we're getting too many, and when either of these happens for long enough, different mechanisms kick in. These mechanisms will either store the extra calories in our fat cells when we're getting more then we need for our day to day energy needs or for releasing these calories out of storage on days that we're not getting enough to cover our energy needs.

Our metabolism and energy levels will change however if we go low calorie for too long (our fat burning efficiency can drop as low as 50%) in 7 days! The reason for this is our survival mechanisms start to kick into defensive mode around the 2nd-3rd day of low calorie intake and within 24 hours of complete fasting.

A low intake of calories for too long will result in our metabolism slowing down to conserve fuel because it detects potential starvation. This process also includes burning muscle for energy needs to slow our metabolism down. Muscle burns lots of calories, and this loss of muscle is why someone has such trouble keeping weight down after a harsh crash diet. Muscle burns calories and much of our metabolism depends on how much we have and how toned this muscle is!

A high calorie meal can be like a Metabolism Reset Button: since our body's fat burning capability starts to slow down around the 3rd low calorie day, (or by the end of a 24 hour fast) I like to think of a cheat meal as simply a way to reset our metabolism back to peak levels!

The way the cheat meal works is simple: our body delivers energy from food to our vital organs and other body tissue necessary for daily function FIRST and the fat cells LAST. Most times after a cheat meal we can feel the food disappear after an hour or so because of the energy deficit we have created by the low calorie days, and this causes our body to suck up these extra calories. When all the cells of our vital and skeletal tissues throughout the body are once again fully stocked with fuel, our metabolism gets really fired up which helps us to burn extra fat over the next few days of calorie restriction!

So after a few days of eating really lean, you don't have to call a binge meal cheating on your diet, but instead it can be called a meal with fat burning purpose!

Our metabolism works a lot like gears in a vehicle: if we learn to shift at the proper time our engine will not sputter so badly and the energy emitted will be much steadier and stronger!

A PALEO DIET

The paleo diet has gotten more attention lately and I believe it is in large part due to the explosion of chronic disease and obesity that seems to be directly connected to our modern day diet.

Paleolithic to me is referring to the era before modern tools, agriculture etc. that had a direct impact on what types of foods were easiest to gather for consumption.

Many of these same people would probably be shaken in their belief system, if they would simply take a trip throughout the human anatomy to really understand why the gastrointestinal track, and the entire human anatomy responds so well to the same foods today that were foods thousands of years ago, such as vegetables, fruits, nuts, seeds berries, eggs, meats from good sources, raw milk and other fermented dairy product. When I took my course in nutrition, I remember thinking of how unsettling this study of the human anatomy and physiology would be to an someone that believes that we evolved from anything less then the hands of a Master Architect that designed the human body to be synchronized with its surroundings and the foods produced there.

 It wasn't until sometime in the past 100 years that having foods from another part of the country or even another part of the world were made possible by super fast logistics by corporations benefitting from cheap foods produced in one area and then sold at a profit to another area, preserved, packaged, processed and convenient to the end user! Back in the Stone Age people were forced to use a more convenient source of groceries, and that meant keeping it local.

These were the hunter, gatherer days, and there was a lot of activity involved in just being able to eat. Fast food back then had the same thing in common with modern fast food in that it was fast and convenient but was a lot more nutritional then the fast food of our era. Death from trauma and infection would have been a much larger cause of death and chronic disease was probably not even considered a risk factor. When you have healthy foods and water (from local sources) combined with steady to high levels of activity it simply helps eliminate chronic disease as a risk factor for death.

We don't have to fully adopt this way of living, it can be as simple as eating a few items listed below everyday combined with some extra activity.

Example foods: vegetables, fruits, lean meats, eggs, nuts and healthy oils. I like quality dairy product as a part of this and (dairy products are a good source of CLA which helps the body convert stored fat into energy). There are many foods that you can pick from in the nut, vegetable, fruit and lean meat categories so that you will always have something around that you like. You can go online and look up Paleo Diet Foods and pull foods from the different categories.

Next on the paleo list: make water the fluid of choice!

Keeping water available and foods that fit in the categories above can help to weed out processed foods, by doing things like eating (nuts instead of a cookie, banana and nut butter instead of a processed diet bar, and water instead of a soda).

Activity: it is important to physically exhaust our pushing, pulling and pressing muscles at least 3 times a week to not only condition our skeletal structure, but also to counter stress hormones. Longer ago when there was stress, there was usually exertion that went with the stress so it helped keep cortisol levels down, (now we oft times are stressed to the max with little physical exertion!)

Note: cortisol is a big contributing factor to belly fat...

We don't have to be radical, but if we gradually fit in new healthy habits, it unconsciously crowds out bad habits and in doing so we will see our health and fitness levels improve and resistance to chronic disease!

POSTURE AND ECONOMY
OF MOVEMENT

When we have a better economy of movement, it makes the things we have to do in daily living easier. And when we can balance our weight properly, it can make our weight or whatever additional weight we are carrying lighter and it will not be as fatiguing throughout our day and will keep from aging our bodies as rapidly. This applies to using proper technique in exercises as well.

In close proximity of our center of gravity, our strength and support goes up, but the further away from this that we get with whatever we're lifting or carrying, the weaker our support system gets.

Example: if you hold a gallon jug of water close to your body, it feels light, but if you hold it out at arms length it will feel very heavy and you will tire rapidly holding it like this. This would get especially tiring if you had to walk a distance holding this gallon jug in this extended position, however if you held it against your body, the load would seem much lighter.

Next try extending your arm out in front of you and walking a distance, eventually your arms would feel like they're supporting a load of bricks compared to when they are hanging along your sides and close to your center of gravity. I'm simply using the above example to show how fatiguing it can be if our body parts are not positioned to make the most of our center of gravity and instead are positioned away from it putting pressure on the back and causing unnecessary compression. Over a period of time this will cause wear and tear much like carrying a load of bricks on one side of a pickup bed, eventually it could cause a degenerative condition on that side or at the least a herniated tire.

Exercise can help strengthen our posture, but we also need to address something else that we do not hear much of and that's muscular balance. This is fairly easy to keep in balance by making so an even amount of exercise is distributed between pulling and pushing exercises. We see this imbalance oft times in someone that puts primary focus on exercises for chest and abs which will eventually pull the shoulders forward because of the amount of muscle on the front side vs. the back side. A good way to check to see if there is an imbalance in strength is to see if you can pull the same amount of weight that you can push.

We can keep ourselves aligned with our center of gravity and improve our posture by keeping our head level with our ear lobes lined up with our shoulders and our shoulders lined up with our hips. This will help with standing or sitting posture and will position us much stronger against whatever weight we carry whether our own bodyweight or additional weight we have to carry. When we keep bad posture, we can expect it to eventually accumulate into degenerative disks, knee and hip problems and at the least miserable bone, joint and spinal conditions!

If we can lighten the load we carry 30%, (by keeping good posture) would it not be worth it, if we were 30% less tired at the end of the day and have 30% less wear and tear on our skeletal structure? This can help us have a much better power and economy of movement in our youth and our Golden Years as well...

MUSCLE AND ECONOMY
OF MOVEMENT

This is one of my favorite subjects because of its effect on pretty much everyone that can still move. A person's economy of movement simply is a measure of how easily they can do their activities of daily living (ADL's) whether an office worker, elite athlete or someone using a wheelchair. Either way the tasks we face throughout each of our day can either be very fatiguing or we can make them become easier by increasing the strength of the muscles that move our tendons, ligaments and skeleton throughout our daily routine, whatever it may be.

Our muscles work a lot like our senses, when we lose one, another tends to become more sensitive helping to compensate for what we lost or don't have.

Example: a person that loses usage of the legs can strengthen upper body muscles to compensate for the lost leg strength or usage, thus increasing the economy of movement and her or his independence.

When we are less active and our muscles become weaker, our weight tends to hang much heavier from our tendons and ligaments causing structural problems and premature aging to our joints. And when this happens, our tendency is to move even less to avoid this pain causing further weakness. If this cycle is not stopped, especially when combined with increased weight gain, the shear weight of our vital organs, body fat, and untoned muscle on our spine, hips, and knees along with the weight of our head on our neck will cause premature aging to our vertebra, joints, tendons and ligaments, causing a degenerative condition to our mobility and eventually causing a dependence on others for our normal activities of daily living (ADL's).

Things we can do: there are lots of exercises that can strengthen movements we use in real life, and you do not have to have a gym or exercise equipment to strengthen functional lifestyle movements. It's as simple as doing the things you have to do oftener and at a faster pace.

Example: if you want to strengthen the muscles you use to go up a flight of stairs, by simply repeating this activity oftener along with a gradual increase in the speed going up the stairs, it will become easier because of our muscles adapting to the new level of stress put on the muscles that help us go up the stairs. This same method works for an athlete as well, and the reason is simple our body is designed to adapt to new or increased stresses.

Isn't it neat that by simply strengthening the muscles that we use throughout our day, can make so we're a lot less tired at the end of our day, making so that we still have the energy for other things and to enjoy the ones we care about?

Strengthening our muscles not only strengthens our movements and makes our days go better; it also takes a lot of weight off of our load bearing joints!

BURNING INTERNAL FAT SNACKS

We have an internal survival system, much like we prepare externally for a time of famine or drought, and when something happens that scares our insides; such as staying hungry for too long or dehydration, it will then prepare itself to protect the body against future stress of this kind.

Example: when we fear a coming shortage of food, we may start simply buying a few extra cans of food (over the amount we normally need) whenever we go grocery shopping. These will simply go into our storage closet or pantry and will be stored there until we have a famine. If we keep adding to this storage for too long and we never have a food shortage or famine to use up what we're storing, our amount of stored food can get out of hand.

When our storage area gets filled up, we have to start looking for new places to store the new food coming in, it's at this point that we start to realize that all this extra food is making our house less functional then it used to be, such as being harder to move around, and when the food that has been stored too long begins to spoil and age it will create a really bad environment inside our home.

Our body's reserve energy storage system works in much the same way in that, it will store the extra food we eat over the amount needed in our fat cells for our use in case we cannot eat. One pound of fat is approximately 3,500 calories and our body goes to this storage area and extracts needed calories when we skip a meal or two.

Fat is often looked at as something we don't like, but it's our body's calorie pantry that our Creator designed to sustain us with through lean times when we need extra calories and cannot access food. This extra fat we have has been a prior investment in excess food intake that we shouldn't feel that we have to go and pay for a bottle of fat burners to be able to burn off.

We can look at the cost of a meal and the amount of calories that it provides, divide and multiply that by the amount of fat we need to lose to measure the amount of investment we have in stored food on our body.

 Example: if we normally eat a meal that provides 700 calories at a cost of $6.00, (there are approximately 3,500 calories per pound of fat) so it would mean that each pound of fat we have extra on our body should be worth $30 in the 5 meals it could provide.

 Each of us has a certain amount of calories that we need on average per day based on what is going on inside us with digestion, body temperature control, vital organs, skeletal muscle, along with our increase or decrease in activities every day. (Our body simply looks for fuel to supply these needs), so if we suddenly drop our calorie intake very low one or two days or skip one or two meals, it forces the body to go to its storage pantry and extract calories.

Example: if your daily need is 2,000 calories and you take in only 1000 calories your body will try to make up this 1000 calorie deficit from your stored energy system.

 You do not want to do calorie restriction like this for too long, or the body will think this is the amount of food it has to get used to everyday, and will simply start burning some muscle to lower its metabolism to become more efficient and not burn calories so fast. Usually if someone skips eating for only 18-24 hours or goes low calorie for 2-3 days and then gets calorie intake back up to regular level, there should be no muscle loss and should result in only in burning fat for energy!

Note: getting blood sugar levels low is the key to unlocking stored body fat and your body's capability to convert it into usable energy, anytime we get a sharp spike in blood sugar, the energy coming from fat storage gets turned off, thus turning off the fat burning process!

FAT WRINKLES

No it's not actually a wrinkle, it's that cellulite we so aggravatingly detect, as we grow older.

Cellulite is to fat as a wrinkle is to skin, it's simply that one is aged skin and the other is aged fat. Though we cannot prevent getting older, there is oft times things we can do to slow down the effects of aging, especially premature aging.

Our skin: when our skin loses elasticity, wrinkles begin to form along with an overall appearance of sagging skin. This can be caused in large part by pollutants our body has to deal with whether in environmental surroundings we are subjected to, or through our food and drink choices.

Our Fat: we have fat cells all over our body; these are backup energy cells to protect us when we cannot eat adequate calories to cover our daily needs. When the caloric intake is not enough to cover our daily need, our body will tap into this supply.

Aging fat: when fat cells are young, the over lying texture is usually supple and smooth, but as we get older we may start seeing some lumpiness aka cellulite. These are unhealthy or aged energy cells (fat cells) that are similar to an aged fuel tank that has signs of rusting and pitting. In the example of car it could come from external road conditions or from external conditions such as bad fuel. This is pretty much the same for our body when toxins are allowed to build up inside causing the cells in our skin, fat and vital organs to age prematurely. Our body is a lot like a factory in that it has toxic matter that needs to be gotten rid of and if we don't get these eliminated properly, they will build up in us and will age the areas it collects in. Not getting rid of these toxins is like putting a lid over a factory's smoke stack, trapping the toxic smoke inside, causing rapid aging to the inside of the factory.

Our body naturally protects us from toxins by either wrapping the toxins in mucous or fat and if these are allowed to build up, we will eventually feel the toxic effects as well as see it in the health of our fat and our skin tone.

What we can do:

1. Increase the antioxidants (fruits and vegetables) in our diet, this gives us much-needed nutrients that help neutralize these toxins that cause oxidative damage to our fat cells.

2. We need exercise to increase circulation and blood flow into these areas to circulate these toxins out of our fat cells.

3. Stimulate circulation with something like a brush that has the little plastic beads at the end and work the area in a circular motion

4. Sweating helps push these toxins out of our body.

5. Increase fiber intake to pull toxins out of our digestive track.

6. Increase water intake to help flush these toxins out through waste elimination and sweating.

Note: whenever you are trying to get rid of fat, or rejuvenate fat for a firmer tone, remember fat cells often accumulate toxins that when released cause oxidation (aging and disease) to other parts of the body they come in contact with, so increasing water intake along with an antioxidant rich diet of fruits and vegetables is important to avoid aging our vital organs, fat cells, and skin!

Doing the above list 1-6 helps us when losing weight to not only look younger as we lose weight but will also help our fat cells to become much healthier energy cells!

Fat is not something we should always think of in terms of how we can get rid of it, but what we can to get our fat cells healthy. Healthy fat under our skin helps us to look younger and healthier as well!

A LIQUID TRAVESTY

Coke is one of the latest but definitely not alone in marketing unhealthy choices to consumers (using a health slant). When these distributors of processed food and drink choices try to hypocritically get into advising the public on healthy choices involving their products, it almost churns my stomach.

If we knew how many people have suffered and are suffering from diseases largely brought on by the bottled, processed drink industry and the billions of dollars profited by them, we would not trust advice on health issues from them or their profit driven motives.

Coke's ad in 2013 seemed designed to counter the public's awareness of the dangers of the toxic aspartame that is used in their diet sodas. Due to falling sales (1% on Coke and 3% on Diet Coke) they want to convince the market that it is okay to consume this toxic sweetener. Rest assured they are not so concerned about our health as they are their falling market share.

 Aspartame is laced throughout so much of our food supply that you can almost rest assured that if its a processed food or drink, you're getting a dose of it, and when its in liquid form imagine how fast it enters the bloodstream and then throughout the body!

 Aspartame has been linked to cancer, diabetes, psychological disorders, slows down weight loss, birth defects, vision problems, brain damage and seizures.

 When there is a chemical that enter the body, it can break down into other more toxic substances, such as aspartame breaking down into DKP, which can produce a chemical that induces the growth of brain tumors. It can also change the chemistry of the brain when the methanol (a component of aspartame) breaks down into formaldehyde, which gathers in areas of the brain causing inflammatory reactions, which can lead to degenerative diseases such as Parkinson and Alzheimer's.

Artificial sweeteners including aspartame products are also bad for our thyroid (this is the organ that regulates our metabolism). These sweeteners are also neurotoxic (nerves and brain) causing an inflammatory response from our body, leading to a release of cortisol, which in turn will signal our body to retain belly fat!

Most other bottled drinks that are not diet drinks are loaded with processed sugars or high fructose corn syrup, and this includes regular sodas, fruit drinks, sweet teas and sports drinks, and when we dump these drinks into our system it can lead to dangerous sugar spikes, which cause obesity and diabetes. Sweet liquid drinks are weight gainer drinks which means when we drink these, (especially when combined with inactivity) we are apt to wear what we drink!

Hydration is next in line for survival behind our need for oxygen, which makes the beverage industry a marketer's dream! When in all actuality, these industries take water (that is naturally ours in the first place), load it up with sugar, caffeine, carbonation, phosphoric acid etc. and then turn back around and sell it to us, marketing it in a way that makes us think it has a higher value then the original base ingredient that makes up the drink...WATER!

God designed our body's makeup with around 60 percent water, (with some vital organs that have a much higher percentage of water), so it's pretty easy to see what we should use to hydrate our body!

The occasional soda, fruit drink, sweet tea etc. is not so bad, it's the habitual drinking of liquid toxins and sugars that causes problems and when combined with inactivity and lack of sweating, the effects are even more toxic!

Do we really want to regularly drink something that contains phosphoric acid (a highly corrosive acid in sodas)? And do we really want to dump a load of sugar and caffeine into our body if the caffeine makes us temporarily insulin insensitive, when we need insulin sensitivity the most?

Will the things that taste good to our mouth feel as good to the rest of my body, or are the desires of my mouth contributing to illness and disease for the rest of my body?

LIGHTEN YOUR LOAD BY INCREASING THE LOAD

This may seem contradictory but it does work when it comes to our skeletal muscle and its capability to adapt to increased workloads and when this increased workload is done regularly over a period of time, it will make the former workload feel lighter.

The exact opposite happens when we become sedentary and our muscles atrophy (shrink) and become weak. When our muscles shrink, movement becomes harder and a greater stress load is put on our bones, tendons, ligaments and joints due to our muscles not supporting the weight we carry adequately. We need to always remember that when our skeletal muscles that help power our physical movements become weaker, our bodyweight will feel heavier and will cause us to tire much easier!

Solution 1: is to do (whatever we expect to be able to continue to do) with consistency. This helps keep things from getting harder, due to keeping the muscles (used for these particular activities) active and familiar with the things you want to be able to continue doing. This works the same way for an athlete that wants to maintain his or her level of capability as well as someone that wants to be able to continue being able to climb a flight of stairs. The best way to be able to keep those stairs from hurting or exhausting us is to continue to use those stairs everyday! This helps keep the muscles used for climbing the stairs, conditioned for this particular activity!

Though solution one above helps us to be able to continue doing our tasks, but it does not make the tasks get easier since our strength only builds up to what we're requiring of it. For this very same reason, if someone keeps repeating the same routine in a exercise routine for a year using the same amount of weight/resistance, a year later it will feel just as heavy, muscle simply adapts to what we require of it.

Solution 2 above: is the one that I really like, since it can help lighten our former load! Its as simple as this example: If you want to make the stairs easier to climb, instead of just taking your body up the stairs, carry some dumbbells up the stairs and carry them back down when you come back. When your muscles get used to carrying you and the dumbbells up the stairs, eventually your weight alone will feel lighter! You can also increase the weight load on your muscles by climbing the stairs faster.

This same principle applies to an athlete or to power-lifting: by simply increasing the load you familiarize your muscle to, over a period of time, will lead to muscle adaption, and will simply make the former load easier on the muscles used for this particular activity.

Example: if an athlete ties a tire to a rope and harnesses it to his or her body and pulls it through the normal track or field exercise, the normal routine or physical demand in the sport will become much easier.

A personal formula to use: think about everything you expect you body to do for you, whether its aggressive in nature such as competitive sports or simply a desire to be independently able to care for your basic needs. Once you know exactly what you expect out of your body, put solution **1** to work and this will help you maintain capabilities, but if you want to make things get easier, start incorporating solution **2** into your routine.

What causes a lot of pain, injuries, and feelings of aging, (is not from doing something the body is used to), but rather something up and beyond what we have conditioned it for. Every so often we need more strength and more endurance, and when our body has been preconditioned, we are less apt to get injured.

If things in life get too easy, we become weaker and eventually even the easy things in life will become harder to do. It's pretty neat to realize that our body is designed to strengthen as a natural reaction during stressful times to guard us against future stresses of similar proportions.

KNOWING THE BASICS OF EXERCISE CAN SAVE YOU MONEY

Over the past 20 plus years of being in the gym business, I have seen a huge industry build up around and profit from over complication of the basics. This can range from someone trying to convince you that an expensive extended personal training package is necessary with your gym membership to commercials touting the latest greatest home gym equipment using a model that definitely used something else (to get in his or her condition) and not what they are paid to help advertise.

There are some simple things to keep in mind to bring balance to any exercise routine, if we don't it can lead to muscle imbalances, blood pressure spikes and dips, along with muscle tightness and loss of flexibility.

There are 5 basic categories to keep in mind when we exercise, whether its using our own bodyweight, exercise equipment or in a gym trying to sketch out a routine from 30 plus pieces of gym equipment. The following is a checklist that in my experience can make it a lot easier for someone that is doing it without a trainer, or to validate your trainer's training techniques.

1. **The warm-up:** this gets your blood warmed up and helps make your veins and arteries expand (vasodilation) and allows for better blood flow to the muscles that you will be exercising. If we start straining on exercises without being warmed up, it can cause a spike in our blood pressure.

2. **The routine(s):** Pulling, Pushing, Pressing. These can be done in one workout or you can split the routine so that you get your various muscle groups at several times per week. Pulling exercises strengthen back and biceps, (such as rowing exercises, pull-ups/ chin-ups etc.). Pushing exercises strengthen chest and triceps, (such as pushups, bench presses etc.). Pressing

strengthens shoulders and legs, (such as overhead dumbbell presses for shoulders and leg press or squats). The main thing to keep in mind is do I have a balanced amount of exercises that I pull toward myself, push away from myself and press away from myself.

3. **Core exercises:** find exercises that not only strengthen your abdominal area but also the lower back, a really good one is the plank. Lie on the floor facing down, raise stomach off floor approximately 3 inches and hold. Weight is balanced on forearms and fore feet. If you are still unclear on this look up "how to do floor planks" on the Internet. This is a back saver that everyone should learn.

4. **Cool down:** the cool down is for the exact opposite of the warm-up. If our blood is really warm and our veins and arteries are still very relaxed and our heart rate slows down too soon after a workout we can get a dive in our blood pressure, you're apt to get very drowsy or you may simply feel your energy bottom out.

Stretch: stretch the muscles worked by stretching them in the opposite way that you were contracting them in the workout.

Learning the above can help you not only in picking the right home gym equipment (or body weight exercises) for your routine, but also helps avoid muscle imbalances and costly personal training fees in a health club. Keep it simple by warming up prior to the workout, do exercises that get your pulling, pushing and pressing muscles, cool down by slowing down but still doing something for the last 5-10 minutes of your workout and then stretch your muscles in the opposite direction of the contractions used throughout the workout.

Exercise, health and fitness are not as complicated as the health, fitness and pharmaceutical industry would have you think.

SUPPLEMENT AND PHARMACEUTICAL FARCE

We look at dietary supplements, and pharmaceutical medicine far too much as a source of health and wellness instead of the things that the above often try to duplicate. Once again, confusion and tactful marketing often convinces us that we need these laboratory created items to burn fat, stay healthy or to get well, when many times by simply adjusting our dietary and lifestyle habits, we can often not only offset the problem but we can also address the root cause of the problem.

Oft times when there is a particular food that helps certain body functions in particular, whether its to release stored fat, use up cholesterol in our blood (to make bile) or lower blood pressure, a laboratory will then try to duplicate this by singling out the main ingredient that causes this effect on our body. They will isolate this ingredient, concentrate it and make it available for purchase to the market so that we can enrich our diet without consumption or extra consumption of the original source(s).

There are a few questions we can ask when considering a supplement:

1. **Am I deficient in this particular nutrient or do I have reason to think that I am deficient?**
   Example 1. A need for protein due to increased demands from physical activities such as sports, physical labor, or exercise routine. Protein powder and Amino Acids help supplement a diet when your intake of meat, eggs, milk, beans etc. is low.
   Example 2. A need for a multi-vitamin-mineral due to a shortage of fruits and vegetables in the diet.

2. **Will I increase these foods in my diet or will I supplement my diet?** We can very easily enrich our diet with almost anything by doing an Internet search for foods rich in this particular nutrient.

Example: if you need more protein in your diet, simply type in "foods rich in protein" or if you

147

need more potassium to lower your need for water pills, type in "foods rich in potassium."

3. **If my decision is to purchase a supplement to my existing diet, do I trust the source/manufacturer?** Quality is very important because if your body cannot properly absorb the nutrient your body will have to figure out how to cleanse it out of the body and if it is unable to, it could cause potential toxicity.

Oxygen, hydration, protein, fat, carbs, vitamins and minerals: are the things we need to supply to our body and we can get these from the air we breath, the fluids we drink and the choice of foods we make for ourselves. Our health largely relies on the quality and balance of these along with adequate activity and rest.

Always remember that supplements are simply a supplement to counter a deficiency in the diet. One reason that foods rich in a certain nutrient can work so much better at supplying this particular nutrient then in isolated supplement form, is all the other nutrients in the food that work together and they understand exactly why they are there and will help each other absorb into the body in perfect unison.

 I have a sheet I like to hand out with a list of over 400 known nutrients that are in an apple, there are many more un-named nutrients in an apple as well! Foods, (especially whole foods) can have over 1000 individual nutrients in them and many times do not work as well when isolated and taken away from their micro-nutrient family.

 We may not know what all these individual nutrients are for or what their purpose is, but they work together and have been created by nature's laboratory that was designed by a Creator who knew exactly how and what it took to supplement our life!

TAKE OWNERSHIP OF YOUR OWN HEALTHCARE SYSTEM

I remember listening in shock to a speech in January of 2003 that president Bush gave on medical tort reform. The reason for my shock was the reason we were given to go to war in the Middle East was to protect Americans over here from terrorism, after a terrorist act that killed almost 3,000 people. I had just heard prior to the speech in 2003, that the 3rd leading cause of Americans dying (around 100,000 per year) was from medical misdiagnosis and hospital infections. "Medical mistakes kill enough people each week to fill four jumbo jets" -Wall Street Journal September 21, 2012.

January of 2003 was my turning point of believing that the war on terrorism was motivated by other things and not so much for the benefit of ordinary American citizens. The next thing I noticed over the past 10 years was a government, media and health reports that were increasingly making our seniors feel insecure about growing old in this country, (whether in their financial or healthcare security.) If someone doesn't show they care about grandma, grandpa, and the unborn, they will not convince me they care about the ones in-between either (except for personally motivated reasons).

When a country's government makes it a critical mission to take over a healthcare system, my opinion is that its for the purpose of making healthcare available, not so much to the ones that deserve it, as for making it available to ones that are of value to them in sustaining the tax system to pay for the debt burden the government is and has been placing on it. And at the same time lowering life expectancy and quality of life for the ones that expect to be able to draw on a social security system they have been paying into most of their life, that our government has been pillaging for the last 25+ years.

There are many passionate doctors, surgeons, specialists and other medical staff (that give themselves unselfishly to the cause and profession they joined) and I don't at all want to sound in a disparaging way toward them, (my uncle is one of these passionate doctors) whether with his patients or on the mission field. The new healthcare laws also catches the medical field in the crosshairs and makes it harder for them to do what they know is best for their patients when its something that falls outside the new guidelines of how they have to treat their patients.

We have however become far too reliant on the healthcare system and should become much more proactive as a country in taking personal responsibility for our own health. I recently had a conversation with my uncle about diabetes and he told me how dependent many patients become on medical treatment while absolutely refusing to make any lifestyle changes that caused this condition in the first place.

Modern medicine has made it possible to address the symptoms on an underlying problem many times without curing the root cause. It's like putting a sump pump in a leaky basement and not concerning ourselves about finding the leak; the problem is that over time the leak is apt to get worse not better! Modern medicine has simply made us way to comfortable with continuing past mistakes that led up to the need of the medicine.

Though advancements have been made in medicine and medical procedures that can seem to extend life or add to the quality of life, we need to ask ourselves a question: what will I do if I can no longer qualify for this procedure or this medicine?

What we can do: we need to take inventory, or an assessment of how dependent we are on anything other then the basics which are; oxygen, water, food, exercise, sunshine and rest? Then ask yourself, why do I have to use this? After we know why we are using something, we need to ask ourselves what is causing the problem? When we fully understand what is causing the problem, it then becomes easier to find a lifestyle change that can address or offset the reason for the medicine, supplement or procedure.

Example: if we have a deteriorating condition in our back, decompressing and then strengthening the muscles in this area can help offset the deteriorating condition, possibly to the point that it relieves this area so much that the body can actually fix it for you!

"Ask why, and ask it again five more times, until all the artifice is stripped away and you end up with the intellectually honest answer"~ Andy Grove

NOT ALL CALORIES ARE CREATED EQUAL

Calories are all measured the same throughout our food system, however the speed at which they enter the bloodstream can make them very different from each other! Some calories are very easily absorbed and their energy becomes rapidly available in our bloodstream without a lot of work on the part of our digestive tract, and is usually from sugary or starchy foods.

Most of the high glycemic or sugary foods that cause these sugar spikes are also the ones that make it hard to lose body fat. This is due to the circulating sugar in our blood, and it locks up the process of burning fat for energy, until the sugar and insulin levels drop back down in the blood. When this happens your body will look for energy to make up for the low blood sugar and can release stored energy from our fat cells thus reducing their size.

Most of the fast absorbing calories are from foods that are either sweet, taste sweet or rapidly brake down into a starchy mush in the mouth. When we eat this, (especially when combined with a sugary drink), it will rapidly enter into the blood, raising blood glucose/sugar levels.

When these calories rapidly enter the blood stream, our insulin will transport them to either working muscle or fat storage and it does this (in order to keep stuff from getting sticky and toxic in all the places our blood goes to). When insulin is not doing this properly, we have what we know as insulin resistance or diabetes. An active lifestyle helps keep blood sugar levels in check and takes a big burden off our insulin-producing pancreas!

It's not always a bad thing to use these fast

absorbing and easy to digest calories, especially when we are going to be physically active after eating these calories. The body converts food into blood glucose for the purpose of supplying energy to working parts of the body and when we get active after eating something that is sugary or rapidly converts to sugars, (such as starches) it allows us to burn these calories off as they enter the blood.

Remember: inactivity after eating (easy to digest calories) causes our body to store this excess spike of calories in our liver and fat cells. And this helps cause a fatty liver and enlarged fat cells!

The above does not apply to someone following an extended period of not eating, such as fasting, our body will rapidly suck up these calories (as long as its not overdone) to feed, refuel and nourish our vital organs and skeletal muscle.

When we eat foods that break down slowly such as dark colored vegetables, beans, lean proteins etc. it helps slow the release of energy into our system and is a much better form of fuel prior to periods of inactivity or very slow activity.

These foods that break down slower also have a higher thermic burn rate then the fast absorbing foods, meaning our body will burn a lot of calories digesting these slower digesting foods!

Example: grilled chicken breast, steamed broccoli, brown rice and beans vs. snicker bar and soda. Even though about an equal amount of calories, the prior will take much longer to digest and will also burn a lot more calories throughout the digestion process then the snicker bar and soda will.

 Kindling is great when used at the right time in starting a fire but it will rapidly fizzle down and die out if not continually fed, but if we use real logs and only use a little kindling to kick start our fire, we will have a constant source of heat and energy that lasts long term.

HOW A MUSCLE CELL GROWS (HYPERTROPHY)

Most of us would like a little more muscle for either, extra strength, shape or simply for better economy of movement or in other words, to have more strength and energy so that whatever we have to do in our daily grind does not wear us out, and that we can have a little steam left to do the fun things in life with the ones we care about.

When our muscle cells expand (hypertrophy) through increased stretch and tension, they simply become stronger, firmer, and have added space inside them to hold more muscle energy (glycogen).

The above is the way our muscle counters and adapts to a new stress placed on the muscle(s) and is also why something that used to be hard to lift, push, pull, press, walk, climb etc. becomes much easier when done consistently and over a period of time, especially when we gradually increase resistance.

Recovery: this is something that is very important to the muscle and strength building process. When muscle cells get put under a stress they're not used to, it causes little micro tears in the muscle and this is what we need nutrition, rest and recovery time to allow our body the time it takes to patch up these muscle cells with amino acids from the proteins in our diet. When our body repairs these muscle cells with this amino acid patch paint creating new protein in the muscle, what we have is a microscopically stronger expanded muscle cell.

It's important to increase these muscle or endurance building stresses over a period of time due to the breakdown process that happens to the muscle proteins in our body. This broken down protein has to be removed (a lot like the waste around a construction site) and if there is too much waste in a short period of time, it can cause things to get clogged up. And in this case it would be an overload on your kidneys! I read recently about a lady's trainer that pushed her way to hard on her first workout and the next morning her urine was the color of Dr. Pepper. She was an insurance agent, and with the type of job she had, her body was probably not close to being prepared for the type of workout her trainer put her through.

Once your muscle is recovered, (usually within 1-2 days) it is ready to be worked again either for the purpose of keeping it at its current strength and size or you can slightly increase the stress to increase strength and muscle size, this depends on your fitness goals. The size of the muscle group worked and intensity of the workout can have a bearing on the amount of recovery time needed.

One of the largest contributing factors to the loss of stamina, strength and performance and the overall aging process is atrophy aka the shrinking of our muscles whether skeletal muscle or the muscles that make up our vital organs and the main 2 factors to this is our diet and inactivity.

Our body adapts to inactivity by shrinking muscle and vital organs (muscle atrophy), but our body also adapts to gradual increases of stress by strengthening our muscle(s) through the hypertrophying of our muscle cells.

Lets live a hypertrophy lifestyle so that our quality of life will not atrophy!

CREATING A STRONGER SKELETAL STRUCTURE

A direct result from an active lifestyle is a stronger skeletal structure along with stronger tendons and ligaments. This also helps stimulate the production of synovial fluid for our joints, which helps them glide more smoothly across each other.

Just like a muscle that becomes stronger (after recovery) as a result from new stresses, our bones become stronger in the much same way. When we exercise with resistance the muscle will pull or push the weight using the bones and joints as levers, guides, and controls, so in actuality muscle in action without its skeletal counterpart would be a pile of useless muscle spasms.

Our body's direct response to inactivity is to shrink things into proportion with our need, this happens with our bones in what we know as bone density. It is a simple process of supply and demand, but it is reduced or increased over a period of time, that is why someone can get skeletal injury or damage when overdoing an activity it is not used to. A gradual increase of stress is how we can get our brain to signal for increased bone density and how our tendons and ligaments strengthen as well.

Chronic inflammatory joint conditions: I like to think of chronic inflammation as an injustice left unattended and the longer it is left to fester, the angrier it gets! This is how our skeletal structure feels if we either gain weight without the supporting muscle to go with it or we are overweight and start becoming inactive causing us to lose the very muscle our skeletal structure is relying on to help split the duty of the carrying this extra weight. Simply imagine a joint area as getting upset with a load it has not been conditioned to carry and we can imagine where the source of the inflammation is coming from a little better. Inflammation is the root source of most all chronic diseases and works in much the same manner in our joint areas, causing discomfort and mobility issues.

Weak bones can be a result of inadequate sun: vitamin D is the sun vitamin and the level of vitamin D in our body largely determines the amount of calcium our body can absorb from our diet. We can have a calcium rich diet, but if we don't have enough vitamin D in our body, it will cause the calcium to pass through unabsorbed.

Exercises for skeletal strengthening: though most exercises will strengthen the skeletal area it tugs against, there are some that we can do that help our joints move in better unison with each other. These are compound movements and are simply real life movements, such as picking a weight off the floor and lifting it above your head, push-ups, pull-ups and squats. Compound movements for a beginner can be as simple as to lay on the floor, (on your back or stomach) and then get back to a standing position; repeat this movement several times. These types of real life movements help muscles, joints, tendons and ligaments to work in synergy with each other. To take it up a notch for increased skeletal strength and capability, simply find a way to add resistance to your selected exercise movement(s).

Our body is unequally designed to continually modify itself for the conditions we place it under;

the weakening or strengthening itself part largely depends on us!

THE BIG FAT DECEPTION!

If I were to pick two words in our vocabulary that have confused and added more to the obesity epidemic then any phrase in our country, it would be the words "Fat Free." When we are trying to lose body fat and we see a food item that looks delicious with the marketing label staring back at us with those words FAT FREE it makes us feel like we're staying on track with our weight loss commitments and goals. These foods are oft times convenient but work directly against what we're trying to do.

Example food mistake: if we were to eat an energy bar with 200 calories it would cause an insulin spike leading to additional fat storage (unless we're active after eating it and doing something to burn it off). If we would take in that same amount of calories in organic butter, it would have an insulin blunting effect, sustained energy (from the fat) over a longer period of time and longer lasting satiety.

Remember: insulin spikes will in turn cause

false hunger signals later even though you have plenty of food in your system.

The problem with these processed ingredients that make these food and drink items taste good, (such as sugar, high fructose corn syrup, and artificial sweeteners) is that they cause our body to have anything from sugar spikes to neurotoxic inflammatory responses that in turn cause us to store fat. Keep in mind the above listed items are put into foods NOT for your health but rather to keep you returning to a deceptive food or drink product that is working against your health and your fitness goals!

Most processed snack foods (diet snacks included) are loaded with these things; this is how they keep their diet items from tasting like cardboard. The key in avoiding these items is to select foods for your diet and snacks that have very few ingredients in them.

Here is what happens with foods and drinks that have added sugar and high fructose corn syrup: when the levels of sugar spike beyond our current energy needs, our body will simply store it for later use, either in our liver or fat cells.

However with artificial sweeteners such as (Sweet n Low, Equal, Splenda) the effect is a little different and may be an indirect cause of weight gain but is a negative effect all the same on our weight loss efforts; they have a bad effect on our thyroid and this is the gland that helps regulate our metabolism. These artificial sweeteners are also neurotoxic causing an inflammatory response from our body, which will cause us to release cortisol, and cortisol is THE stress hormone that causes us to retain belly fat!

Keeping it simple works best: only eat or drink sweets before or right after long or intense periods of activity, avoid food or drink products with artificial sweeteners or high fructose corn syrup.

Most times fat is not the problem, an over abundance of starches and or sugars in our diet is the real culprit. However when high fat foods are consumed in combination with sugary foods or drink the fat can be a problem because of the spike in insulin due to the sugar intake.

When we learn what real food and drink is, we can spot the foods that are wasting our time in our health and fitness efforts and when we truly visualize how much these foods and beverages are working against our efforts, they will not taste or look so good!

FAT CLUMSY LIVERS

This organ is responsible for over 500 crucial functions, SO THIS IS SERIOUS! Non alcoholic fatty liver disease (NAFLD) wasn't even an issue 30 years ago, now it affects as many as a 3rd of us in America and is the leading form of liver disease in the United States!

One of my members recently had blood work done and was telling me how surprised the medical staff was that he had no signs of fat accumulation in his liver. She said that most people they test at his age (44) either have or are showing signs of a fatty liver.

A fat liver is unable to perform as well as a lean healthy liver, and since our liver helps with so many critical functions of the body, this can become a major generator of various health issues and symptoms whether to us personally or throughout our healthcare system.

Why is this so big a problem? I believe to find this out, we need to simply look at what we are doing differently that is causing our liver to store more fat.

The sugar trap: I've been researching something that I like to call a sugar trap, which is simply sugars/glucose that gets trapped in our blood by insulin resistance. Insulin resistance can be caused by huge surges of insulin from eating high sugar food and drink over a long period of time. It can also come from caffeine, which causes temporary insulin insensitivity. Either way when the cells of our body are not receptive to insulin (which is our sugar transport agent) and these sugars are left trapped in the blood for too long, it can really cause problems, imagine how sticky and syrupy things get if these sugars stay in the blood. This can slow down circulation, which can cause blindness and amputated limbs due to the lack of circulation. These trapped sugars also cause advanced glycation end products (AGE's) that cause rapid aging.

High fructose corn syrup: this sweetener is especially bad since it breaks down much easier because of the fructose/glucose ratio is not 50/50 like sugar, its a 55/45 ratio of fructose to glucose and it's this easy to break apart binding, that lets it slide like quick silver into our bloodstream without the normal breakdown in the digestive track or the spike in insulin which is our sugar digestion hormone. If this fructose is not burned off while in the blood, it will rapidly go to the liver and trigger lipogenesis, which is the process in which the liver converts the fructose to blood fats.

Opinion: I believe our body is designed to reroute things when it's necessary to protect us and if this is true our body will be looking for a place to deposit these extra sugars that we are not burning off. If we have insulin resistance, (even if temporarily from caffeine consumed with sugary foods), it only makes sense that trapped fructose and glucose circulate to the liver, where the liver attempts to store it as a defense mechanism not to hurt us but simply to keep blood glucose levels safe.

Once these extra unburned, unabsorbed sugars get transported to the liver, it will go through a conversion process where the liver changes sugar over into fat through a process called lipogenesis and triglyceride synthesis. It then becomes a stored energy in the form of fat. This is an awesome way for our body to control the uptake and the release of energy, however if our liver is constantly taking up energy and not releasing it in equal proportions, it only makes sense that it will continue to build up in our liver and our network of blood vessels.

What we can do: the reserve energy in our liver is a primary source for an energy snack when we go into a calorie deficit, so if we simply cut our calorie intake down to about half of our normal daily intake for 1-2 days, this decrease in calories will cause your liver to release reserve energy snacks (fat) back into the blood in the form of triglycerides.

Opinion: I believe that creating periodic calorie deficits will help decrease the fat in our liver in the same way calorie deficits will cause the release of energy inside our fat cells throughout our entire body for their calorie content thus making them smaller fat cells.

Our liver is our largest solid state organ handling 500+ crucial functions in our body, and when it is able to properly perform, just imagine how efficient our inner healthcare system can become when a network of 500+ functions is affected by a healthy liver that not only breaks down and helps get rid of our body's toxic waste products, but generates energy and nutrients for our body as well!

YOU'RE NOT EXPECTED TO OUTLIVE YOUR PARENTS

For the first time in the history, the younger generation is not expected to outlive their parents. When I first heard this years ago, I thought it meant that if we don't change our habits and the habits of our children that this would happen, however, we are seeing this happening all around us now. This has been a source of inspiration to me ever since in doing what I can to create awareness.

This has been heavy on my heart and mind this week especially because of a long time friend of mine having a massive stroke on Monday. My friend Mike was only 40 years old and is part of a growing statistic of young people that are suffering from or have died from stroke. Right now one-third of stroke victims are between the age of 20 and 64 and this number they say could double by 2030. I woke up this morning and almost as soon as I turned on the news they were discussing the alarming growth of young people having stroke. And standing there with my friend's dad in the ICU Tuesday evening and my friend unable to speak or move his right side has shown me how personal this epidemic is apt to become to most of us.

There are two things to consider: potential genetical weaknesses and simply chronic disease our lifestyle may have incurred. Both require changes in lifestyle to either change what we are doing to ourselves or to strengthen ourselves against genetic weaknesses.

Example: heart disease has prevailed itself several times on my moms side of the family, so the chances are greater that this could be an underlying problem for me personally. However a lot of what is going on with the explosion of chronic disease in the generation ages (30-60) is directly related to our lifestyle and probably a perfect storm of things that are different then they used to be.

What we have to look at: though heart disease, stroke, cancer and diabetes are the main culprits, we have to address what is feeding these fires, things like how our food and drink choices have changed, how ingredients in these foods and drinks are chemically altered, and also how our activity levels have changed when they majorly should have increased to offset the effects of these food like products. What can we do to put ourselves in better control of the above?

We also need to look at how quick we are to medicate and then become satisfied with the results our medications give, so we stay on them so that we do not have to make the lifestyle changes that led us up to the need of the medicine in the first place! What lifestyle change can I make to reduce or eliminate my need to medicate this symptom(s)?

What we can do: I like to imagine taking up healthy dietary and exercise habits as being like a mechanic hooking up a radiator to a flushing system and as this flushing system circulates the new fluids through the system, the rust and sludge gradually releases until only clean fluid remains and when this happens the cooling system runs much more efficiently as well as the systems that it protects.

Doing periodic intermittent fasting (IF) to lower body and blood fats, and doing periodic 4-7 day system cleanses using a combination of antioxidant rich vegetables, fruits and nuts (mostly raw) along with plenty of activity/exercise to sweat out and to help rid our body of toxins should help speed up the process of cleansing and resetting our body's systems.

If anything, this past week (seeing what my friend is going through) has made me a lot more appreciative of mobility and for having been blessed with good health so far. I do believe that no matter how healthy we think we are this can be taken away from any of us either by death or a debilitating illness or disease, however we should be good stewards of what God has blessed us with and I believe God will bless our efforts. Even though each of our days may be numbered, our concern should be in having a longer health span and not so much our life span...

We cannot put bad fluids into our vehicle, or leave it parked too long without increasing the chances of sludge building up and gaskets getting brittle and hard thus affecting its performance or the life of our engine and the body that it powers.

EXERCISE MONITOR

We monitor and record many things throughout our life for such things as maintaining or bettering work performance etc. It would probably help if we used the same approach in our exercise routine and other higher output activities in our life. As with most anything whether mental or physical, it takes maintenance to keep you at a certain level and increased conditioning to take you further.

Our body keeps a certain level of strength by a consistent routine and strengthens itself further based on increased demands our routine or activity level asks of it.

Example: walking up and down hills instead of a flat stretch, carrying a set of dumbbells up and down a flight of stairs instead of just your bodyweight.

A friend of mine recently was telling me about a house that he and his wife bought that they consider the last house they plan to purchase, in other words they plan to grow old in it. He said a friend told him a house with an upstairs may not be good once the children leave because of having to go up and down stairs (this is where I stopped him) and said this is exactly what you need to have as you get older. I told him he should make so that something is upstairs that he and his wife need to go to almost daily, such as an office or something. This will consistently condition the muscles they need to get up and down the stairs. When a person quits doing an activity or certain activities, the muscles associated with these movements lose their size, tone and strength.

One of the primary things that contribute to muscles atrophying (shrinking in size and strength) is lack of activity and lack of restricted activity such as in resistance training exercises. This is largely the reason a person gets so tired when they do something they haven't done in a long time or something they haven't been conditioning for through exercise.

Example: if my friend would quit going up and down the stairs and after a few months would decide to carry some boxes up the stairs for storage, (besides potentially putting his back at risk for spinal compression and inflammation) it would be much more exhausting due to the muscles used having lost their tone.

The reason it's so important to have physical things we do regularly (whether exercising in a gym or our own home routine) is to measure our current capabilities against our future needs. This includes, upper body, core and lower body conditioning.

Example: it's really easy for us to keep tabs on our strength and fitness level by doing a few basic exercises. We primarily have (pushing and pulling muscles in our upper body and the muscles throughout our core and lower body that we use to do a squatting exercise) throughout our skeletal system and if we have a few exercises that hit these particular groups we can monitor our strength levels. We can also monitor our endurance level by going from one muscle group to the next.

Example home strength and endurance routine: do a set of pushups, next do a set of squats, next do a set of bent rows, next see how long you can do a floor plank, rest and then repeat

Example gym strength and endurance routine: do a set of bench presses, next do a set of weighted bar squats, next do a set of cable rows or lat pull-downs, next see how long you can do a floor plank, rest and repeat.

Record your performance: resistance, speed, time then measure how many heartbeats per minute.

 Whether its muscle strength, muscle tone, muscle size, or muscle and cardio endurance, our body prepares for tomorrow by what we subject it to today!

WHY MANY SUPPLEMENTS ARE B.S.

Bowel Secretion is our body's way of flushing things it doesn't need or that it doesn't recognize, and there are many supplements on the market that find their way into the sewer system and if our body rejects them, its probably a good place for it to be, rather then staying in us and causing toxicities.

Americans spend over $11 billion per year on dietary supplements and this amount is expected to grow to $15.5 billion by 2017. This is a big business and as in years past you will see a lot of hype designed for these companies to get their market share in this lucrative business.

Our body was designed to absorb and process nutrients we need through whole food and whenever it gets processed foods or supplements that have ingredients in them that it recognizes as toxic to the body, it will separate them from the things it does recognize and will try to move the toxic ingredients out through one of our body's elimination processes. If it is unable to eliminate these toxic ingredients (whether it be in processed food, vaccines, environmental, medications, supplements etc.) and if these toxins continue to build up, it can trigger an inflammatory immune system response. And a continued inflammatory response (chronic inflammation) is the source of most all chronic disease and chronic joint conditions.

Supplements are simply for replacing nutrient shortages in our diets and if we don't have a shortage of a particular nutrient the body will oft times eliminate it through our waste. When we have a balanced diet, our body can pick through thousands of nutrients to get what it needs to keep in balanced, however if we are not getting adequate amounts of something in our diet, we can add in a supplement to help make up the difference.

How to know you need a supplement: there are several ways to figure out what is missing in your diet, we need macronutrients (proteins, fats and carbs) and we need micronutrients (vitamins, phytonutrients and minerals). If we are not getting any one of the above fairly regularly, we may notice a difference in our energy, strength, recovery, bone density and immune system. We can also have a blood profile done to see if we have nutrient deficiencies.

Reasons you may need a supplement(s): if you do not get enough fruits and vegetables in your diet, you may need a multivitamin or a fruit/vegetable powder mix. If you are very active in sports, exercise and the activities of daily living, you may benefit from protein or amino acids for muscle recovery. If you don't get much dairy or calcium rich plant foods you probably should supplement at least occasionally with calcium and vitamin D.

There are quite a few supplements on the market now that research has advanced and they're great at helping bridge the gap between what we should be getting in our diet and what we're actually getting, BUT we need to make sure that the product has at least a few credentials that checkout before trusting it enough to put it inside you!

How to find good supplements: you can checkout most reputable companies online, their background, scientific research on products, and years in business. The thing that I rely on the most (for my source of multivitamins and minerals) is years of scientific research. I also like staying a minimum of six months behind the curve after a new product is developed to give myself time to see positive or negative feedback.

Good quality food is always your best bet and a good way to get a balance is to find out which foods belong in each category, and then make so you eat something from each group throughout the day and have a variety to choose from throughout a 7 day period. The main thing is to keep your blood nutrient levels healthy with the variety of nutrients your body needs to maintain maximum health.

Dietary supplements are simply designed to supplement a diet that is lacking in this particular nutrient(s).

Keep it simple: your body needs protein, fat, carbs, vitamins, minerals and phytonutrients, if you feel like you're not getting adequate amounts from one group, you may benefit from dietary supplementation. Last but most important; research the company and the product.

 To say that a dietary supplement is equal to another because it has the same supplement name is like claiming that a hamburger from Krystal's is the same as one from Five Guys Burgers, just because they're both burgers.

HOW BEANS CAN LOWER YOUR CHOLESTEROL

Its active ingredient for this process is simply the large content of soluble fiber beans (and other soluble fiber rich foods) contain and the process is simply the removal of bile through the stool which causes our body to have to produce more and it makes the new bile from cholesterol. The main thing to remember when it comes to the difference between this fiber and insoluble fiber is that soluble fiber is or becomes a jelly like substance and slows absorption of fats and sugars and insoluble fiber stays fibrous and helps keep old food debris from clinging to the walls of our digestive track and colon walls.

In 2014 changes were made to make a lot of our population qualify for statin drug treatment. It will double the amount of people being able to qualify for the glorious honor of receiving statin drugs for their cardiovascular conditions. This news report made me feel like I was about to spit nails!

STATINS ARE THE MOST PRESCRIBED DRUG IN THE HISTORY OF MEDICINE and the most profitable. In 2012 they were a $26 billion dollar industry and these new guidelines could effectively double this!

One of the new guidelines is for ages 40-70 that have a 7.5% risk of developing cardiovascular disease would then be able to qualify for statins. My question is this; if the number one killer of Americans is heart disease, wouldn't this 7.5% risk factor pretty much qualify everyone as a statin drug client? This is a cholesterol medicine but the new guidelines are also calling for consideration of the persons overall risk factor and not so much whether or not they have a cholesterol problem.

SIDE EFFECTS OF STATINS: the required warnings from the FDA include, risk of liver damage, memory loss, confusion, type 2 Diabetes, and add to this list the potential of muscle weakness, joint pain, COQ-10 depletion which in turn causes lower cellular energy levels which can also weaken the heart pump in patients with heart failure.

How soluble fiber works: soluble fiber becomes a gel like product that slows down absorption of fats and sugars in our digestive track, (this is why sugar from fruits is absorbed more slowly then factory processed sugar products). Our gall bladder sprinkles bile over fatty foods we eat to help break fat. The soluble fiber makes so it's not as easy for our body to reabsorb the bile back up to the liver (from our digestive track) and then back out to the gall bladders storage tank. When we lose bile through our stool it forces the liver to have to make new bile salts and the main ingredient that our liver uses to form new bile salts is CHOLESTEROL.

If we can mix in more foods rich in soluble fiber (especially when eating fatty foods) and lower our intake of starches and sugars (other then the sugars from fruits) we should have an effective cholesterol lowering diet.

List of foods rich in soluble fiber: kidney beans, black beans, navy beans, oatmeal, brown rice, apples, bananas, prunes, citrus fruits, Brussels sprouts, green leafy vegetables, sweet potatoes. When in doubt add BeneFiber or Metamucil with your meals. This is pretty much tasteless soluble fiber so it can be mixed into low fiber foods or water and is a good way to help increase our soluble fiber intake.

Benefits of a cholesterol lowering diet: helps control cholesterol, lower the risk of diabetes, high blood pressure, coronary artery disease, obesity, hemorrhoids, colon cancer, constipation and irritable bowel syndrome (IBS, all without the side effects of statin drugs.

If we would look at statins and other awesome modern medicine as a temporary fix instead of a long-term solution these medicines would serve their purpose much better. Oft times these high powered medications lead people to believe they don't have to change the lifestyle that led up to the need of the medicine in the first place.

In keeping with Hippocrates' famous saying, "Let thy food be thy medicine and let thy medicine be thy food," just as selecting the right medicine for the ailment is necessary to hit the nail on the head, we need to increase our soluble fiber intake to help lower or keep our cholesterol in check or we will very possibly become a future statin drug customer.

IMMUNE STRESS + REST
= IMMUNITY

The equation above is the same as physical conditioning with workouts, "Workout stress + Recovery = Increased Strength and Conditioning."

Without the above formula being used, we can expect an increased chance that we will become weakened and potentially injured.

We are going into the flu season and it's something that we usually get anxious about every year, (whether for ourselves or our family) and we hope the bug will pass over us. What we don't realize is that many times we may come in contact with the bug and it may actually get to set on our shoulder for a little while before we finally shake it off.

The above is our innate immune system at work, this part of our immune system is the one that silently goes to work killing the bad and warding off viruses and infections that oft times we don't even know were trying to invade.

Just like exposing our muscles to a good workout regularly helps keep them conditioned and strong, our immune system also needs to be exposed to viruses, germs and bacteria to keep it strong and if we try to live in a sanitized bubble with no germ or virus exposure guess what??? WE WEAKEN OUR IMMUNE SYSTEM!

When we finish a really hard workout, even though we may not feel it yet, our body has been weakened temporarily by the workout even though there are some immediate physiological benefits. However, if we give our muscles adequate rest, these same muscles that were broken down by straining harder then they were accustomed to will come back stronger then before. They will also carry out heavier tasks without straining as much (because of muscle adaption). Our immune system works in almost exactly the same way. If we go around trying to sanitize everything, trying to make sure that our immune system is never exposed to anything, (just like our muscles adapting to inactivity by getting smaller and weaker), our immune system will also get weaker due to no activity.

I believe besides diet, one of our biggest mistakes after being exposed to the flu virus or being injected with the virus (vaccination) is not getting adequate rest afterwards so that our body can redirect its energy into fighting off the invader(s).

Whether we have been vaccinated for synthetically building our immune system or we come in contact with a person(s) that has a virus, (and especially during flu season) we should listen to our body and if we start feeling fatigued at unusual times, we should decrease external activity so that our body can direct the energy toward the inner battle it is trying to fight.

Try to remember: whenever being exposed to a crowd where your immune system may be put to task in the days following, listen closely to what your body is saying. When suddenly you get extremely tired, try to rest instead of stubbornly pushing your way through whether by will power or stimulants. When we keep pushing ourselves, our body will eventually put us down so it can start the recovery process!

Diet: drink lots of water (it's important to stay hydrated so that our body can flush the bad things out that its trying to get rid of). If you feel you're a little dehydrated, put a pinch of salt in the water. Eat foods that fuel your immune system, but keep foods light and easy to digest; soups and other soft foods such as chicken and noodle soup are great. Digesting heavy foods takes a lot of energy, and keeping food intake light and steady helps nourish it without sucking up a lot of energy that your immune system needs. This does not include drinking lots of sugar loaded fruit juices.

A strong immune system stays in good condition by exposure and once exposed will create a memory of the bad things it came in contact with. This memory is stored in our innate immune system and it will create the exact tools needed to silently execute future encounters like your own personal team of ninjas!

CALORIES AND COLD TEMPERATURES

Feeling a blast of winter air probably has most of us doing something to get warmer or to stay warm. The neat thing about cold weather and our body is its own way of heating itself. Cold can crank up something called cold thermogenesis and it can actually help us burn fat through heat generation!

We have a pea-sized thing in our brain, called the hypothalamus and it is our body's thermostat, regulating many other things but a big part of this is regulating our body's temperature and a lot of our body's required daily calories are for the purpose of temperature control.

Calories are units of heat and are to temperature control in the body as fuel is to a fire. And stored body fat is to this process like stored logs are to heat a house during times of gas or electric shortage (through the regular power grid or energy source).

Fat storage: when we have a shortage of fuel in our stomach and digestive tract, our body will go to our storage units (fat cells) to release calories/units of heat.

Shivering: is a way that our body generates heat as well, through this process will generate heat back into our body and works pretty much opposite of our body's cooling system where it pushes excess heat out of our body.

A lot of the reason many of us experience appetite increases during the winter is because of our body having to build a bigger fire to heat itself. We can use these times to force our body to pull calories (units of heat) from our storage areas (fatty deposits) by dropping our calorie intake for 1-2 days. What our body doesn't get through our digestive tract it will simply pull from our fatty deposit areas, whether liver or more visible areas around muscle and under the skin.

Example: if your daily calorie requirement is 2300 calories and you only get 1000 calories through that day's food intake, your body will go to your storage areas and release calories from the fat cells, and in this example would need to release approximately 1300. There are approximately 3500 calories in a pound of fat.

Our winter diet should consist of foods higher in fat and protein and much lower in starches and sugars. It makes sense to me because like throwing fuel on a log fire may cause a spike in heat, it will be short term and will not be conducive to creating a good steady long lasting heat source. Also it's a lot easier when you're already using a certain type of heat source to stay with this same fuel as the primary source.

Example: it would be like having your regular supply of wood beside the fireplace, but if you run low you can simply carry some in from your porch or other storage area attached to your house.

If we use our excess energy properly during the winter, when spring and summer comes around we won't have to worry about so much excess fat and just like extra logs left unused for too long, will become pitted and old, our fat can also start looking aged in the form of cellulite!

HOLIDAY CALORIE FURNACE

Most of us have probably successfully store more calories then we would like to over the holidays, but then most of us probably didn't intend to under eat at the events scattered throughout this festive time of year!

There are two things that usually seem to happen during the holidays:

1. An increase of calorie intake.

2. A decrease in intense physical activity.
When we have a decrease in physical activity but an increase in caloric intake over an extended time period, it simply tells our body to store this energy until later in our fat cells and fatty deposit areas.

MUSCLE IS OUR BODY'S CALORIE FURNACE!!! The more you have of it and the more toned and conditioned it is, the hotter your thermogenic (fat burning) fire will be! We too often relate a decrease in metabolism to aging, but it's not nearly so much the aging factor as it is a decrease in quality muscle mass. And the two primary causes of this is our decrease in physical activity and our diet! These two factors coincidently are the two main contributing factors in the aging process as well.

Boosting metabolism and slowing the aging process are some really good reasons to add extra muscle and strength to your life, especially when combined with better joint health, mobility, and a better looking shape!

When we build muscle there are three stages that increase the pace that our body burns calories:

1. During exercise (working muscles need fuel)

2. Recovery (our body has to move nutrients to broken down areas for the recovery process and in building stronger muscle)

3. The added muscle burns extra calories at the pace of about 13-16 calories a day per pound.

Keep in mind that the first two months of a good exercise program and diet increases a lot of muscle weight, while decreasing the fat weight so oft times we do not see a lot of scale change until after the

2nd month. Its usually by the 2nd month, muscle we already have, has toned up, so it's not unusual for a person to gain 8-12 pounds of muscle while losing 12-15 pounds of fat in the first two months. This means that some will only see a 3-pound decrease on the scale for all this effort. The reward is in the increased muscle strength, increased metabolism and a better shape!

Building muscle while losing fat, keeps us from having the shrunken balloon syndrome and appearance. When we let some air out of a balloon, with nothing to replace it, the balloon gets a saggy and older looking appearance. This is also why a person may look better and healthier at a larger size.

If you want to increase your body's natural capability to burn off fat and extra calories, the answer is in toning and building muscle and not in expensive fat burners that boost a fake metabolism. Age is not an excuse either; you can tone and build muscle at any age!

Our body knows how to release calories from stored fat as a food and energy source without fat burners and expensive diets; it can even make its own drugs for illness, infection and disease! To do these powerful and complicated things, our body only wants the simple things...

I wish you all the best in health & Fitness!
Wade Yoder

About the author

Wade Yoder has been in the health and fitness club business since 1991 and is a weekly health and fitness columnist for 5 Middle, Georgia newspapers with over 160 published articles since 2012.
He owns and operates Valley Athletic Club in Fort Valley, Georgia

Master Trainer certifications:

Fitness Trainer - Fitness Nutrition

Fitness Therapy - Strength and Conditioning

Senior Fitness & Youth Fitness